Keto for Women Over 50

Why it's not too late to lose weight, burn fat, and prevent the most common signs of aging.

Includes 21-Day meal plan, simple recipes, and everything about Keto you need to know

written by
Tracy Pedrini

Table of Contents

Introduction

The ketogenic diet has soared in popularity. However, it is not a new plan or idea; the ketogenic diet has been around for a hundred years. Rather than the many popular fad diets, you see in magazines, the ketogenic diet was created by teams of doctors, has been used in a number of scientific studies, and was created for the purpose of improving health. Because of this, you can trust not only your ability to lose weight with this plan but also your ability to gain benefits for your health as you age.

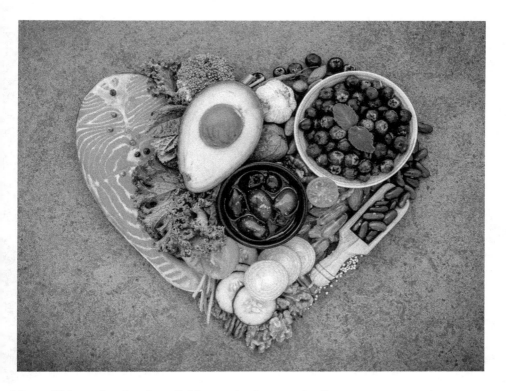

You will love the food available on the ketogenic diet, as you can enjoy a number of delicious ingredients. Foods such as avocados, bacon, butter, cheese, and nuts are all available to you. But even if you choose to avoid meat or dairy, you can still enjoy this plan with other sources of healthy fat. With the number of delicious foods available, you will find that it is easier than ever to watch your weight while maintaining an active and fun social life. You can still enjoy eating out with friends and family while knowing that you are watching your waistline and caring for your health.

In this book, you will find everything you need to gain the weight, health, and lifestyle you desire and deserve. You will learn about the basics of the ketogenic diet, the science behind the plan, the difference between good and bad fats, a step-by-step guide to beginning the plan, recipes including ten dessert recipes, a 21-day meal plan, and more!

Chapter 1: Keto Diet 101

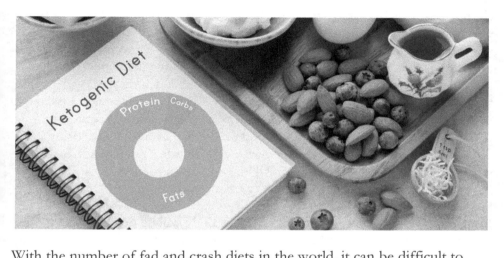

With the number of fad and crash diets in the world, it can be difficult to know what to turn to when you need to lose weight or improve your health. Whether your reasons for choosing a diet are to reduce the size of your weight line, lower your blood pressure, or reduce your blood sugar, you will find that the number of diet options is astounding. Yet, many of these popular diets are not healthy, as they promote unmaintainable rapid weight loss that results in malnutrition. As these diets are unmaintainable, you will eventually fall off the wagon, and the yo-yo effect on your metabolism will only cause you to gain more weight than you ever lost. Sadly, this pattern results in many women steadily gaining weight over the years as they try one crash diet after another. Thankfully, there is a different option available. You don't have to punish your body and mind to lose weight. There is a way you can lose weight and promote health in a maintainable way. The answer? The ketogenic diet. With this diet, you can limit the number of carbohydrates you eat and instead replace them with healthy fats and protein. There is no specific calorie count or points you have assigned, as each person and their needs are different. All you have to do is find the number of calories your individual body needs and eat plenty of protein, fat, and low-starch vegetables to attain your personalized goal.

You don't have to take my word for it about the powerful effects and benefits of this plan. The ketogenic diet has a long and robust history and scientific backing proving its effects. In this chapter, we will touch on the history and the basics of the diet, and in the next chapter, we will discuss the proven science.

Many of the popular crash and fad diets today were thought up by people in Hollywood as a way to quickly lose weight, even if it was not maintainable. Companies will also capitalize on these fads by creating products or entire programs to sell people, making them millions every year. Yet, while companies are making all of this money off of peoples' attempts, it often only causes frustration on the part of individuals. While many people lose a lot of water weight the first week on the ketogenic diet, after that, weight loss becomes more slow and steady, which is good! Think about weight loss as the race between the tortoise and the hare. The hare might have made progress much more quickly, they ended up getting worn out and losing in the end. On the other hand, the tortoise worked at their own maintainable pace, allowing them to cross the finish line and reach their goal. Studies have long shown that weight loss works in the same way.

If a person loses weight overly quickly, their body will be unable to keep up. It is not only unmaintainable, but it is also a sign that your body is under too much stress or being deprived of important nutrients. The result? You may lose weight quickly at first, but you will either damage your health in the process or gain even more weight later on when your metabolism snaps back like a rubber band that was pulled too far.

By losing weight slowly and steadily, you can ensure you nourish your body, giving it all the nutrients you need and increase your health in the process. You can also promote your metabolism instead of harming it, meaning that you will not experience a weight yo-yo in which you put on even more pounds than you initially lost. While we all may idolize the hare, we should all aim to be more like the tortoise, instead.

Believe it or not, the ketogenic diet first took root in the treatment of epilepsy and other neurological diseases. This is good news, as it means that you can receive many neurological health benefits such as improved memory and more. We will cover these health benefits in a later chapter.

In 1911, researchers and doctors in France ran a study on the effects of fasting and epilepsy. This study found that when a person fasted, they experienced fewer seizures. Although researchers would not discover why until years later, it was due to the production of ketone bodies when a person fasts. This study inspired similar studies and treatment of epilepsy in the United States shortly thereafter, especially by Dr. Hugh Conklin. By treating his patients with long-term fasting, Dr. Conklin was greatly able to improve the neurological health of his patients, especially those who were adolescents.

The studies on fasting's benefits on neurological disorders continued, despite one main problem: fasting is not maintainable long-term. But, researchers sought ways to overcome this obstacle, and a short time later, Dr. H. Rawle Geyelin discovered the answer. Dr. Geyelin discovered that if a person ate a low-carb and high-fat diet, they could receive the same benefits without fasting. This allowed participants to eat all the nutrients their body required and enjoy food while still allowing them to reduce their seizure activity. While this diet would later become known as the ketogenic diet, it was still not named at this time as researchers had yet to discover ketone bodies that give the diet its name and benefits.

After completing a study with thirty-six patients on his version of the ketogenic diet, Dr. Geyelin reported his findings to the American Medical Association. The ketogenic diet was a great medical discovery and began to take the medical world by storm, which leads to many researchers across the world conducting their own studies and doctors prescribing the diet to their patients with epilepsy.

The ketogenic diet first began to gain nationwide awareness outside of the medical community in the '90s. At this point, ketone bodies had been discovered, the ketogenic diet had been named, and it was largely understood by doctors. However, while the ketogenic diet had been popular in the past, it had waned in popularity for a time due to the invention of anti-seizure medication. Due to the creation of these drugs, doctors believed for a time that the ketogenic diet was unnecessary, as they believed a pill could help more than any diet. Yet, anti-seizure medication is not helpful for every patient, and it can cause drastic side effects. The limits and side effects of anti-seizure medication lead to a renewal in the use of the ketogenic diet for epilepsy, which would later lead to it being used more widely for other health conditions and weight loss.

In 1994, Dateline aired an episode featuring the Abrahams family, who had tried every option of anti-seizure medication available for their son Charlie. Nothing worked and Charlie's condition only continued to worsen, so his parents began to research on their own. No doctor had recommended the ketogenic diet since, at this point, it was still believed to be inferior to medication. But, after reading through a medical journal, his parents discovered the ketogenic diet.

There was only one hospital in the country that was still using the ketogenic diet to treat patients: Johns Hopkins Hospital. Charlie and his parents traveled to go see Dr. John Freeman, who was overseeing the use of the ketogenic diet at Johns Hopkins. Soon after Dr. Freeman began to treat Charlie, his health progressed rapidly. He experienced a drastic decrease in seizure activity and his developmental growth, which had been stalled, began to get back on track, all thanks to the ketogenic diet. While no drug had ever helped Charlie, the ketogenic diet changed everything.

After having such success with the ketogenic diet, Abraham's family wanted to spread knowledge and awareness to help other people with epilepsy. Not only did they appear on Dateline to achieve this, but they also started the Charlie Foundation, and Charlie's father, Jim Abrahams, produced a movie telling their story. This movie starred Meryl Streep and was titled First Do No Harm.

Now that you have a basic understanding of the history of the ketogenic diet let's look at the two main basic principles behind the plan: the macro ratio and micronutrients.

The Macro Ratio

The macronutrients are found within everything you eat, as they consist of protein, fat, and carbohydrates. On the ketogenic diet, there are certain ratios of these macronutrients that you will eat, known as the macro ratio. Most of these ratios are about the same, but there can be some varieties. The reason that there is not one set macro ratio for everyone is that every person is different. Some people may need to eat a larger serving of protein due to their activity level or size. Since every person has their own ideal caloric intake level, their fat intake will be matched to their personal needs. Carbohydrates are most regularly the same, with most people consuming up to twenty-five net carbohydrates daily, although this can vary, as well. Let's look at the macronutrients each in turn.

It is vital that a person tracks their macronutrients and knows their macro ratio, otherwise, they can run into a number of problems. For instance, since fats are high caloric, a person may accidentally eat too many if they aren't tracking them, which can lead to stalls in weight loss. However, a person can run into many other problems if they don't track their macros, as eating too little protein can cause muscle wasting and weakening. Thankfully, it is easy to track your macros, as we will cover in a later chapter.

Protein:

The human body needs a certain amount of glucose to feed certain cells, such as brain cells. However, this does not mean you need to eat carbohydrates. In fact, carbohydrates are the only type of macronutrient that humans can survive and thrive without. This is because the body has a way to generate its own glucose by transmuting protein in a process known as gluconeogenesis. Yet, while protein and fats are necessary for human survival, there is no way for our bodies to replicate these fuel sources, which means we must consume enough of them in our diet.

The amount of protein you eat on the ketogenic diet is the most important so that you can maintain muscle health, energy, and brain health. Every person's protein needs will vary, sometimes greatly, but it is generally around twenty-five percent of a person's food intake. You will be able to find your specific protein needs by using a macronutrient calculator.

There are many different types of protein you can enjoy on the ketogenic diet. This includes fish, poultry, red meat, shellfish, eggs, dairy, seeds, nuts, and low-carb soy products such as tofu. Keep in mind that these products are not pure protein, and they will contain a certain amount of the other two macronutrients as well. This means that if you eat one slice of cheddar cheese (111 calories), you can't simply count all the calories in the cheese toward your protein intake. Instead, you will have to calculate all three macronutrients in the cheese. Let's have a look at the macronutrients in this slice of cheese and how they each affect the total calorie count:

- Protein – 7 grams = 28
- Fat – 9 grams = 81 calories
- Carbohydrates – 0.4 grams = 2 calories

As you can see, each of the three macronutrients makes up the total calories. You can easily calculate how much a given macronutrient affects your daily macro ratio by reading the nutrition label on food and knowing how many calories are in a given macronutrient. Fat is the highest in calories with 9 calories for each gram of fat. Both protein and carbohydrates have 4 calories per gram. Of course, while you can calculate this on your own, you don't have to. Later on, in this book, I will provide you with a number of resources that will track your macronutrient intake and goal for you, which takes the work out of staying on track.

Carbohydrates:

All carbs are not created equal, which is something important to understand on the ketogenic diet. What does this mean? Well, if you look at certain nutritional labels (not all), it will have a category for both total carbohydrates and net carbs. The difference between the two will drastically change the number of carbs you can eat in a given day and still stay in ketosis.

A single cup of 2% milk contains 12 grams of total carbohydrates. Dairy, especially milk and low-fat varieties of cheese, is a high carbohydrate food. But, it is also low in certain other nutrients, such as fiber.

On the other hand, a cup of almonds contains 20 grams of total carbohydrates. It may seem that the cup of almonds is higher in carbohydrates than 2% milk, but this is not fully accurate. The reason for this is because almonds are also high in fiber, containing 11 grams of fiber. While fiber is a form of carbohydrate, it is not digested by the stomach. Instead, fiber slows down digestion to allow our bodies to fully absorb the nutrients, and it is then expelled from the body. The result? We don't need to count the fiber in our daily total of carbohydrates as our bodies are not digesting them. When you extract the grams of fiber from the total carbohydrate count, you are left with the net carb count. In this case, the net carbs for one cup of almonds are 9 grams. Some foods sold under the label "low-carb" will label the net carb count for you. However, most products don't list specific net carb counts, so you will have to calculate it yourself by removing the number of fiber grams from the grams of total carbs. It is a super simple process and only takes a moment.

Along with fiber, you can also remove carbohydrates from sugar alcohols out of the equation to determine an ingredient's net carb count, as sugar alcohols are also expelled from the body without being digested. The two most common sugar alcohols that this applies to are erythritol and xylitol, which are frequently used in low-carb sweeteners.

Many people on the ketogenic diet will avoid fruits and vegetables due to their carbohydrate content, but this is not healthy. Remember, produce contains vital vitamins, minerals, and phytonutrients that the human body needs to stay healthy. Sure, you may prefer to eat your entire net carb ratio for the day in cheese, it is more important to make room for several servings of vegetables. Thankfully, there are many low-carb vegetables you can enjoy! It is best to have some knowledge of net carb counts in the vegetables you eat, but if you are unable to look it up online, you can always choose a low-starch variety. For instance, potatoes are high in starch which results in a high net carb count. On the other hand, broccoli is a low-starch vegetable, and thereby, low in net carbs.

You can still enjoy cheese, bacon, and nuts on the ketogenic diet, just make sure that you also include a few servings of vegetables a day. Some vegetables are even high in healthy fats, such as avocados and olives, although olives are technically fruit.

Many fruits are high in carbs due to their natural sugar content, but there are some fruits you can still enjoy in moderation. The best choice of sweet fruits are berries, which are not only the lowest-carb options but also some of the highest in nutrition.

You will be surprised how many things contain carbohydrates, which is why it is so important to track your net carb intake. Carbs frequently hide in dairy products, nuts, seeds, vegetables, and other everyday foods. It is best to avoid milk, low-fat dairy, starchy vegetables, most fruit, cashews, and pistachios. These all have higher net carb counts than they are worth and can throw off your nutrition for the day. For instance, even if you eat a small enough number of cashews to not go over your daily allotment of net carbs, it will still take up so many carbs from the rest of your day that you are unable to eat well. Instead, choose lower carb options, such as almonds. Similarly, foods that are high in carbohydrates, such as grains and beans, should be avoided completely. The only exceptions are green beans, which are a low-starch vegetable, and soy products that have had most of the carbs removed, such as tofu and soy milk.

Fat:
While there is often a specific percentage or number given for carbohydrate and protein intake (25 net carbs and 25% protein), the amount of fat a person might eat varies greatly. This is because a person needs a specific amount of protein to maintain health and no more than twenty-five net carbs to maintain ketosis. But, since everyone needs a personalized caloric intake, the way we can vary the number of calories we are eating is by customizing our fat intake. This means that one person might eat 1,000 calories worth of fat, whereas another person might eat 2,000 calories worth of fat. If you want to customize your weight goals, then all you have to do is alter the number of calories of fat you eat. For instance, you can eat exactly your daily recommendation of calories to maintain weight, a reduced-calorie count to lose weight, or even an excess of calories if you need to gain weight.

There are many sources of fat that you can choose from, but ideally, you want to minimize unhealthy fats while prioritizing healthy fats. We will discuss fats in more depth in a later chapter.

You might worry about increasing your fat intake, but keep in mind that fat does not make you fat and all fats are not created equal. Yes, unhealthy fats might worsen heart health, but on the other hand, studies have found healthy sources of fat improve both heart and brain health. Similarly, carbs are much more likely to make a person gain weight and bloat that fat. The misconception that fats make a person fat is due to fat being more calorie-dense than carbohydrates and protein. But, as long as you ensure you are not eating more fats than you should for your daily calorie count, then you will continue to lose weight.

The Micronutrients

On the ketogenic diet, many people focus on their macronutrients but forget about their micronutrients. What are micronutrients? These are nutrients that your body needs in a smaller number than macronutrients, but that equally as important for human health. Any vitamin or mineral that humans require counts as a micronutrient.

When a person is busy and used to eating a lot of junk food, they can fall into bad eating habits, even on the ketogenic diet. When this happens, whether on the ketogenic diet or the standard American diet, a person tends to eat less nutritious food (such as vegetables, fruits, nuts, seeds, etc.) leading to deficiencies and malnourishment. Because of this, you have to be sure that whether you are on the ketogenic diet or not that you prioritize healthy ingredients and that you eat a variety of vegetables daily. Don't just depend on your favorite high-fat foods like bacon, cream cheese, and cheddar cheese. Include plenty of asparagus, broccoli, spaghetti squash, green beans, cauliflower, radishes, and bell peppers. Eat a moderation of almonds, chia seeds, flax seeds, macadamia nuts, olives, and avocados.

While you should get enough micronutrients by eating a balanced ketogenic diet, there are certain micronutrients that people are more likely than others to become deficient in if they do not eat a balanced keto diet. We'll delve into these specific micronutrients so that you can ensure you eat enough of each.

Sodium:

While society is largely aware of the dangers of too much sodium, aside from athletes, not many people are aware of the dangers of too little sodium, also known as salt. Yes, an excess of salt can cause heart disease, high blood pressure, and many other conditions. But, salt is also an essential mineral and electrolyte for human health. To put it bluntly, without salt, a person would die.

Just as too much salt can negatively impact your heart health, too little salt will as well. This is because the electrolytes, such as salt, allow your muscles to contract and your nerves to communicate with each other. Without this ability, your heart would no longer be able to pump blood through your arteries and veins.

Many people have only had to worry about an excess of salt in their diets, but when you begin the ketogenic diet, it is important to be aware that you may have to make an effort to get enough sodium in your daily life. There are multiple reasons for this, but the biggest one is that when you enter ketosis, you will lose excess water weight. This water weight is water molecules that were attached to the carbohydrate cells in your body. But, when you go on a low-carb diet and no longer have an excess of carbs within your system, then your body has no reason to hold onto excess water and will dump it through your urine, causing the standard water weight loss we are all familiar with. The problem with this is that electrolytes are stored within these water molecules, and when you lose water weight quickly, it results in a rapid loss of vital electrolytes, including sodium.
You may also lose sodium later on in the ketogenic diet if you have insulin resistance. This is because insulin resistance causes a person's body to hold onto excessive sodium. But, the ketogenic diet treats insulin resistance getting your insulin response back to a healthy normal. As this happens, your body will no longer be holding onto its excessive stores of sodium, and if you eat only low-sodium foods you might not get enough.

Thankfully, most people only have to worry about sodium deficiencies during the early stages of keto when they are losing water weight, and it is easy to fix. All you have to do is ensure you drink plenty of water and liberally salt your food. Doctors generally recommend for adults to eat between three and five grams of sodium daily.

Some symptoms of sodium deficiency include muscle spasms, headaches, dizziness, nausea, vomiting, fatigue, confusion, irritability, restlessness, muscle cramps, and muscle weakness.

Potassium:

Another electrolyte, meaning it is used for muscle contraction, nerve cell communication, and heart health is potassium. Many people think that if you need more potassium, you have to eat a banana, but you will be happy to know there are many low-carb sources of potassium, some of which have much more than a banana!

You can become deficient in potassium due to the same reason as sodium: you lose water weight too quickly. When this happens, you may not experience any symptoms, so it is a good idea to ensure you are eating plenty of potassium in your diet regardless of symptoms. However, this doesn't mean symptoms never occur. Sometimes, people experience irritability, constipation, weakness, muscle loss, skin disorders, irregular heartbeat, or heart palpitations.

In general, doctors recommend adults consume forty-five hundred milligrams of potassium daily. Some options for high-potassium foods that are keto-friendly include avocados, kale, spinach, and mushrooms.

Magnesium:

A third of four of the electrolytes is magnesium. This is one of the most versatile of our electrolytes, as it plays a role in over three hundred biochemical functions within the human body. If you don't have enough magnesium, it can negatively affect your body's ability to produce cells, manage energy levels, form important fatty acids, or synthesize protein.

Sadly, many people do not consume enough magnesium in their diets, leading to magnesium deficiencies being common and widely under-diagnosed. People experience fatigue, dizziness, and muscle cramps, with no idea that these symptoms are caused due to a lack of magnesium. Thankfully, there are plenty of ways you can increase your body's magnesium supply, and you don't even have to eat it.

You can get more magnesium in Swiss chard, pumpkin seeds, and oysters. But, you can also add magnesium salt, known as Epsom salt, to your bath water, use muscle pain relief gels that contain magnesium, or take supplements. These other ways work, as magnesium is readily absorbed through the skin.

Calcium:

The last electrolyte and the one people are most aware of the importance of is calcium. But, while people know the importance of calcium, there are many misconceptions. For instance, milk is not the best way to get calcium. In fact, the calcium found within dairy is largely ineffective. You would do much better-consuming calcium in the form of broccoli, kale, almonds, and bone-in sardines than in dairy products.

Along with being important for bone and teeth health, calcium also helps with nerve cell communication, maintaining proper blood clotting when injured, and managing blood pressure. In general, doctors recommend at least twelve hundred milligrams of calcium daily for women over fifty.

Chapter 2: The Science Behind the Plan

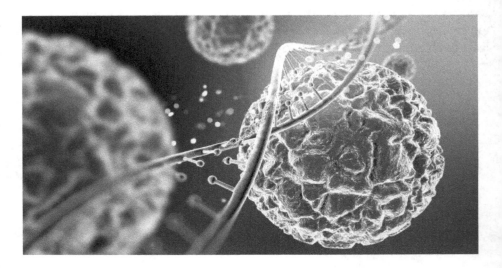

The ketogenic diet has many benefits. It can help people with chronic illness and disease, it can encourage weight loss, and when customized, can help underweight people gain weight. But, that is not all. Due to the science behind the principles of the ketogenic diet, it can specifically help women who are over fifty to lose weight and gain health. In this chapter, we will briefly explore the science in an easy-to-understand and fun manner so that you can have absolute faith in knowing that you are making the best choice to care for yourself.

You may have heard that the ketogenic diet can increase your metabolism, but most people only have a vague idea of what their metabolism is and how to utilize it. Before getting into the how of ketogenic metabolic increase, let's explore what metabolism is and how it can be used to benefit your health and weight.

Put simply, the metabolic process, otherwise known as your metabolism, is your body's process of ingesting food, transforming it into fuel, and then burning that fuel to create energy for the body. The metabolic process is keeping your body alive and thriving on a moment-by-moment basis, whether you are awake or sleeping. This metabolic process allows your heart to pump blood through your veins, your lungs to take air in and out, your cells to stay alive and functioning, and it manages all your other biological functions. Monitoring your weight, whether through weight gain, weight loss, or weight maintenance, is only one small aspect of the metabolic process.

Every person's metabolic process works differently, which can especially be seen in how a person gains or lose weight. For instance, one person may be able to eat high-caloric food all day long and still struggle with being medically underweight. On the other hand, a person may eat a balanced and generally healthy low-calorie diet, despite struggling with being medically classified as overweight. Every person's metabolic process will work differently based on their genetics, age, and more.

For women over fifty, age can greatly affect their metabolism. Even if they were at a standard weight their entire lives, they may begin to struggle with increasing weight gain. This is because many peoples' metabolism will slow down as they age. The older you get, the slower your metabolism will become.

When a person's metabolism becomes slower with age, it means that their body burns fewer calories, resulting in more fat being stored within the body's cells. This change in metabolism can make it difficult to lose weight, even if you reduce your caloric intake. Thankfully, the ketogenic diet can help you overcome this, boost your metabolism, and work with your aging metabolism to help decrease stored body fat.

The human body contains over thirty-seven trillion cells. It is hard to even comprehend this number, as it is larger than anything we can imagine. But, every single one of these cells plays a vital role in our body, which we can not survive without. The ketogenic diet is able to help a portion of these cells excel in their duties. The mitochondrial cells are a special type of cell that contains mitochondria, a component of the cell that allows them to break down any fuel source into energy, whether it is amino acids, fatty acids, glucose, or ketone bodies. By decreasing carbohydrates, we are thereby decreasing the fuel glucose, and in the same way, by increasing fat, we are also increasing the fatty acid fuel. This change in fuel sources gives the mitochondrial cells the healthier fuel sources they crave, allowing them to become healthier, work better, and thereby increase their metabolism.

While some cells within the human body can only survive with specific fuel sources, the mitochondrial cells are different in that they can utilize any type of fuel source. But, this does not mean all sources of fuel are created equal. For instance, when the mitochondrial cells are forced to use a large amount of glucose for fuel, it causes dangerous toxins and oxidants to be released into the body. These oxidants and toxins are well-known to increase aging and our risks of developing diseases as we age. But, by replacing your glucose fuel with fatty acids, you can decrease the oxidants and toxins, thereby improving your mitochondrial and overall health.

But, what about the non-mitochondrial cells that require glucose? Thankfully, glucose, while needed by some cells to function, is the only fuel source the human body does not need to ingest. We must eat fat and protein to produce fatty acids and amino acids for fuel. On the other hand, when we do not eat carbohydrates, our body can produce glucose specifically for the cells that require it through the process of gluconeogenesis. This process does not produce excess glucose, meaning your mitochondrial cells will not utilize the glucose; they will still rely on healthier fuel sources. But, the cells that require glucose (such as brain cells) will have the glucose they require to survive. This gluconeogenesis process works by converting excess amino acids in the body into glucose, giving your body the amount of glucose it needs and no more, maintaining a perfect balance. This balance is achievable when on the ketogenic diet, as you are eating the ideal balance of fuel sources for your body.

When a person is not on the ketogenic diet, and they are eating a standard Western diet full of carbohydrates, the mitochondrial cells are unable to utilize the healthier sources of fuel, such as fatty acids. This is because glucose is a fast-acting fuel source, and the mitochondrial cells will automatically prioritize the use of any fast-acting fuel source, even if there are other healthier fuel sources available.

But, this is not all. The human body is only able to store so much glucose at one point. Most adults are only able to hold up to twelve hundred calories of glucose within their muscles and liver at a given moment. But, if you have more glucose than this within your body, what happens to it? Since the human body is unable to store more glucose than this, it is forced to convert the excess glucose into body fat, also known as adipose tissue. To avoid having to convert the glucose and then store it as fat, the mitochondrial cells must first burn off the glucose for fuel before using the healthier fuel sources. This means that if you limit your glucose intake on the ketogenic diet, you can also decrease your stored body fat and increase the number of healthy fuel sources your cells can utilize.

When on the ketogenic diet, not only do the mitochondrial cells receive the benefit of utilizing amino acids and fatty acids instead of glucose for a fuel source, they also receive an additional non-ingested fuel source: ketone bodies. The fourth fuel type, ketones, is produced within the body, but only when a person has a low level of glucose within their cells. This means that most people don't regularly produce ketones, as they eat frequently ensuring that they always have a fresh supply of glucose. On the other hand, on the ketogenic diet, you prioritize eating low-carbohydrate foods, allowing your body the chance to produce ketone bodies, which are a superior fuel source.

These ketone bodies are largely what give the ketogenic diet its benefits, after all, the "keto" portion of the name is derived from the word "ketone." The entire ketogenic diet is based around these ketone bodies and the benefits they produce. For instance, it is these ketone bodies that allow the brain to protect itself from seizures, dementia, and old age.

But, if ketone bodies are superior, why does the body only produce them on a low-carb diet? As you know, some cells require glucose for fuel. Most of these cells are brain cells, but the kidney medulla, red blood cells, and testicle cells all also require glucose. Generally, the body will use the process of gluconeogenesis to convert amino acids into glucose for these cells. But, in order to utilize less glucose, the process of ketosis begins to convert fatty acids into ketone bodies. The benefit of these ketone bodies is that, unlike fatty acids, they can cross the blood-brain barrier and be used as fuel by cells that typically only burn glucose. This is beneficial, as glucose releases harmful toxins when burned as a fuel source, but ketones do not. The result is that by using ketones as fuel instead of glucose, you can protect your brain health as you age, staying more mentally agile and reducing your risk of age-related diseases. The longer your body utilizes these ketone bodies, the more benefits you will experience. You may not be able to physically see these changes, but your body will feel them. Your body's inflammation levels will lower, you will experience more energy, sleep better, and find that your body's hunger cravings balance out.

Chapter 3: Good Fats vs. Bad Fats

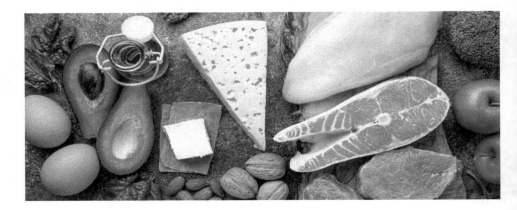

The ketogenic diet is low in carbohydrates and high in fats, which means that you need to understand the difference between good fats and bad fats. If you don't understand this difference, it would be all too easy to eat unhealthy fats, leading to degrading health and increased cholesterol levels. On the other hand, if you prioritize healthy fats, you can lower your cholesterol, lose weight, and increase your overall health. Many people have experienced these benefits, and doctors have been amazed, but to experience this, you must have this basic understanding. Thankfully, once you learn the basics of only a few fat types, you can easily prioritize the best fats while limiting other options, ensuring you get the highest quality experience on the ketogenic diet.

The Best Sources of Fat

There are several types of high-quality fat you can choose from on your daily keto diet, which makes it easy to ensure you get plenty of the good stuff and little of the bad. As you have a variety of choices, you can ensure that you never get bored, as you have many flavors and ingredients to choose from. While you may choose to prioritize one or two of these top fat choices, when possible, it is a good idea to enjoy a variety of all of them, as they each have their health benefits.

Fish:

Fish are not only a great source of protein, but many types of fish are also high in micronutrients and healthy fats. Salmon is most known for this, but there are many other options, as well. For instance, sardines are an ideal source of healthy fats. Not only are they just as high in omega-3 as salmon, but when they are eaten bone-in, they are also higher in calcium, and as they are a smaller type of fish, they are lower in toxic mercury.

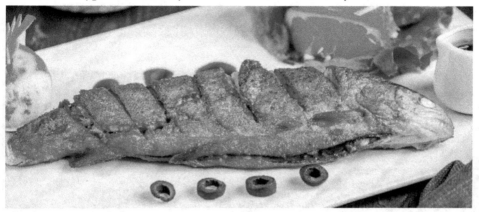

Keep in mind that many people do not consume enough omega-3 fatty acids, causing an imbalance in the omega-3 and omega-6 ratio, resulting in inflammation and a number of potential health risks. Therefore, it is best to eat fatty fish at least three times a week, prioritizing smaller fish to limit your mercury intake.

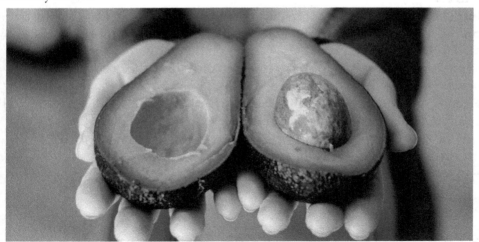

Avocado:
Avocados are frequently thought of as vegetables, but they are a fruit with a rich source of healthy fats. This is good news, considering how popular they have become in recent years. Not only can you find avocados and guacamole in most grocery stores, but you can also find avocado oil, salad dressings made with avocado oil, and other keto-friendly products filled with this healthy fat.

Avocado is largely made up of monounsaturated fats, known as MUFAs. This is a heart-healthy fat type that decreases inflammation, lowers bad cholesterol, raises good cholesterol, and is ideal for cooking even at high temperatures. When you eat the avocado fruit, you even get the added benefit of fiber, micronutrients, and phytonutrients.

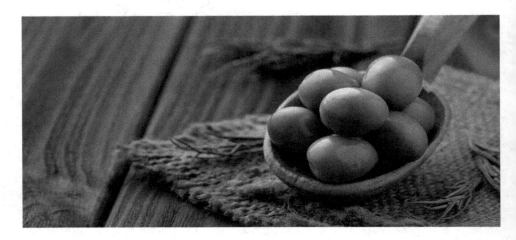

Olives:
Just like avocados, olives are frequently thought of as a vegetable but are a fruit high in some of the healthiest fats around monounsaturated fats. This means that just as avocados and avocado oil can lower your cholesterol and improve your health, so too can olives and olive oil. When using olives, it is best to use high-grade extra-virgin olive oil, as any olive oil classified as "light tasting" or "extra light" contains decreased health benefits. While avocado oil excels in cooking at high temperatures, olive oil does better cooking at low and moderate temperatures or being served raw in the form of salad dressings or drizzling over your meal.

Nuts:
Whether you are eating nuts in their whole form, as butter or as oils, there are many health benefits. The best two options are whole nuts and nut butter, as these contain the full fiber and phytonutrient contents. On the other hand, nut oils don't contain fiber or phytonutrients, but they also don't contain any carbs, meaning you can add them to your ketogenic diet more easily. Thankfully, you don't have to choose one or the other, you can include a

balance of all three nut fat types in your ketogenic diet to receive all the benefits you could hope for.

Some of the best nut options to choose from on the ketogenic diet include almonds, walnuts, pistachios, pecans, hazelnuts, and macadamia nuts.

Peanuts are a legume, not a nut, but they have their benefits in moderation. Just keep in mind that many peanut products have added unhealthy fats, sugar, or other additives. When choosing peanut products, it is best to choose natural peanut butter without added fats or sweeteners.

Brazil nuts are a great source of fat and micronutrient, selenium, but due to their high selenium content, they should only be eaten in extreme moderation so that you do not consume too much of this mineral. A single Brazil nut can provide an adult with their daily selenium recommendation.

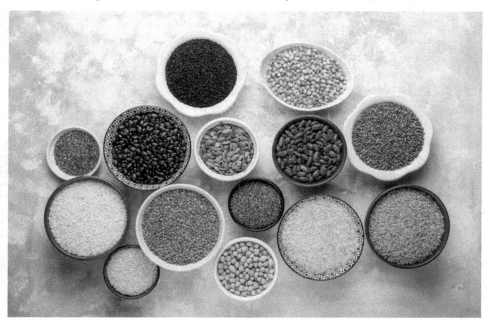

Chia Seeds and Flaxseeds:
These two seeds are two of the best plant-based sources of omega-3 fatty acids. While the human body is unable to process plant-based omega-3 fatty acids in the same amount as animal-based, there are still many benefits to consuming these two seeds. Along with being full of healthy fats, these seeds are also full of protein, fiber, micronutrients, and phytonutrients. They can lower cholesterol, reduce insulin resistance, reduce the risks of diabetes, and decrease obesity. Whether you enjoy these seeds in their whole forms, as oils, or as supplements, you are sure to receive many health benefits.

Another bonus of these two seeds is that they can be used to make many low-carb treats, both sweet and savory.

Moderate Quality Fats

The fats in this category are frequently eaten in high numbers on the ketogenic diet. But, if you eat too many of these fats, you may find that your cholesterol levels rise. However, that is not to say that these fats don't have their health benefits. The fats in this category have both pros and cons, and therefore, should be enjoyed in moderation, with a higher priority placed on the fats in the previous category.

Butter:

Dairy-sourced fats are, as a general, not the best for your health. In high numbers, they can increase your cholesterol and cause a domino effect of other poor health results. But, that is not to say that dairy-based fats are whole bad, either. In fact, grass-fed butter, such as the brand Kerrygold, contains quite a few important vitamins. While regular butter you find in the store contains very few nutrients, due to the diet of grass-fed cows, this butter contains five times the nutrient density. Grass-fed butter is also full of vitamin K2, which is an important vitamin difficult to find in any other source. So, you can enjoy your butter in moderation, but when you do, try to choose higher-quality brands, such as grass-fed Kerrygold. You will find that it is worth the switch, as it is not only higher in nutrition but also in flavor. Once you try it, you won't go back!

Cheese:

Just like butter, not all cheese is created equal, as it largely depends on the quality of the diet the cows were fed. When purchasing cheese, it is best to choose high-quality cheeses that are higher in fat, as low-fat and skim milk cheeses contain more carbohydrates. Cheese is also a great source of protein, making it a good way to get a healthy snack when you are feeling low on energy. But, avoid using cheese in every meal as some people are prone to do on the ketogenic diet. Remember, the fats in this category are to be enjoyed in moderation.

Cream:

Heavy cream is a great way to add some more fat and calories into your diet, and you can use it as a replacement for higher-carb options. For instance, instead of using milk in your coffee, you can use heavy cream or half-n'-half. When choosing a cream, it is best to shop around and try to find grass-fed varieties. It may cost more, but it will be well worth the switch for your health and the flavor. To get grass-fed cream, you might need to shop at a health food store, such as Whole Foods, or search for your local dairies.

Remember, heavy cream from cows is not the only option! You might be able to find a local farmer selling goat's cream, sheep's cream, or even other types of heavy cream. Cream from any of these animal sources will do, as long as the animals are fed a high-quality grass diet.

Fats to be wary of

The fats found within meat and milk, known as trans fats, are enjoyed on the ketogenic diet, but you really should keep these in moderation. Milk should be especially avoided anyways, as it is high in carbs, and therefore, not keto-friendly. Some people on the ketogenic diet make the mistake of eating a breakfast of nothing but bacon and cheese. This is not a healthy breakfast, as not only is it low in micronutrients, but it also contains the types of fats you should keep in moderation instead of the healthiest fat choices. Instead, you would do better eating an omelet with avocado, mushrooms, spinach, a slice of bacon, and a serving of your favorite cheese. As you can see, with this breakfast, you are still eating bacon and cheese, but you are enjoying them in moderation and paired with healthier ingredients for a full and balanced meal.

When you do eat meat on the ketogenic diet, you can eat higher fat meats such as bacon and beef, but you should balance them out with low-fat options such as poultry. By choosing lower-fat options, you can optimize your protein intake while minimizing your trans fat intake. This way instead of simply eating bacon or high-fat ground beef, you can enjoy a richly seasoned chicken breast paired with an olive tapenade, guacamole, or a toasted nut coating. By balancing your meals in this way, you get the best fats and the best sources of protein, optimizing your health and the flavors in your meal.

What about Coconut Oil?

There are pros and cons to coconut oil. For instance, this fat, especially when its purified form and sold as MCT oil (medium-chain triglyceride oil) can help reduce the risk of dementia and Alzheimer's disease, which can increase metabolism, reduce belly fat, decrease hunger, and decrease the risk of heart disease. However, coconut oil is saturated fat, which isn't the best source of fat. This means that you can receive health benefits from coconut oil and MCT oil in moderation, but in excess, you may begin to experience adverse effects. Some people will eat almost entirely coconut oil as a fat source, but this may lead to increased cholesterol rather than decreased cholesterol.

Therefore, you should balance out your coconut oil intake along with other healthy fats, such as olives, avocados, nuts, and seeds.

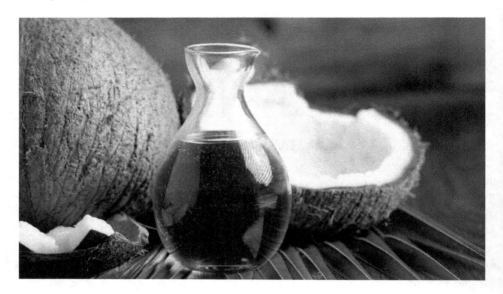

Many nutritionists are warning their patients about coconut oil. Not because coconut oil is a terrible fat, but because many people misunderstand the benefits of coconut oil, and therefore, don't realize that it should be eaten in moderation. Coconut oil is not the perfect fat, and in excess, it won't help you. Remember, maintain moderation and balance in all aspects of your ketogenic diet if you want to experience all the health benefits it has to offer.

While studies have found that people in cultures who eat a large amount of coconut oil generally have lower cholesterol than those that do not, this is not only due to coconut oil. These cultures often frequently eat other healthy foods, such as olive oil, nuts, seeds, fish, and vegetables; along with a much lower number of heavily processed junk foods or sugar than those on a standard Western diet.

Studies have found that in these cultures that eat a large number of coconut products, those that eat the highest amount of coconut-based fats also have the highest levels of bad cholesterol out of these groups of cultures. Remember, you can't contribute an entire culture's health levels to a single ingredient, as many various aspects go into a culture's health.

In a series of eight clinical studies, the effects of coconut oil in a person's diet was compared to both butter (a saturated fat, like coconut oil) and olive oil or safflower oil, which are unsaturated fats. These studies found that coconut oil raised harmful cholesterol more than unsaturated fats. However, it also found that coconut oil generally does not raise cholesterol more than saturated fats such as butter, palm oil, or beef fat.

This means that you can enjoy coconut oil and its health benefits, but just as you should limit your intake of dairy and red meat, you should also limit coconut oil. It is not fat you should be scared of, but you also shouldn't eat all coconut oil. Instead, prioritize the fats mentioned in the first section of this chapter, and supplement your diet with coconut oil to maintain a healthy balance of all your choices.

Chapter 4: The Health Benefits

There are many health benefits of the ketogenic diet, and these benefits can apply to a wide range of individuals. But, what many do not realize is that many of these benefits specifically help women fifty and older. In this chapter, we will explore how you can improve your health and weight with the ketogenic diet, decreasing your risk of disease as you age and increasing your vitality.

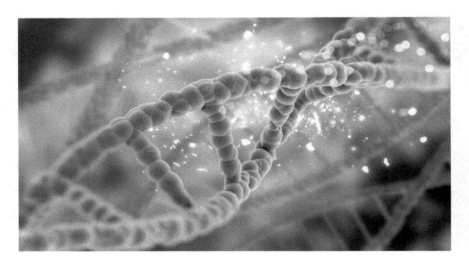

Preserve Your DNA

One way the ketogenic diet can help women as they age is by affecting the chromosomes. These chromosomes are structures within our DNA, with two dozen being found within each of our cells. At the end of these chromosomes, structures are the telomeres, which act as a form of shielding and protection for the chromosomes. The telomeres ensure that the chromosomes stay healthy and strong. However, as we age, these telomeres can shorten, increasing our risk of developing age-related diseases.

While the chromosomes and telomeres may be indecipherable to the naked eye, there are still ways we can increase their health and preserve their strength. Studies have found that our diet can greatly affect the length and health of our telomeres, and therefore our chromosomes, as well. While some foods may degrade the telomere and increase our risk of developing high cholesterol, heart-related diseases, or diabetes, other foods can have the opposite effect. Many of the foods that you are encouraged to eat on the ketogenic diet have been found to preserve the telomere, therefore, decreasing a person's rate of aging and decreasing the risk of diseases.

One stunning example of food affecting the health of telomeres is the study between the risk of diseases and the consumption of nuts and seeds. Studies have found that when people eat a higher percentage of nuts and seeds, as is encouraged on the ketogenic diet, people experience stronger and healthier telomeres, live longer, and experience better overall health.

This same study also found that highly processes meats, such as Spam and bacon, resulting in shorter and weaker telomeres. The more processed foods a person eats, the more their chromosomes and telomere will degrade, resulting in increased aging and decreased health. What does this mean? While you can certainly enjoy bacon in moderation on the ketogenic diet, it is important to focus on eating natural whole foods that have not been heavily processed.

Foods that can increase telomere strength and health are typically high in healthy fats and protein while being minimally processed. Some great examples include:

- Organ meats
- Olive oil
- Avocados
- Macadamia nuts
- Shellfish
- Fatty fish
- Non-hydrogenated animal fat
- Egg yolks
- Butter
- MCT oil
- Nut butter

Increase Energy

As we age, we naturally lose energy. While it might have previously been easy to work a full-time job and then go partying through all hours of the night, as we get older, we find that just doing what we have to do gets exhausting. But, there are ways we can increase our energy. By changing your diet, you will find that you have the capabilities to not only do more but feel better while you do it.

You have most likely heard the phrase "you are what you eat," your entire life. While this phrase may not be literal, what you eat does become the fuel for your cells, which then affects how you can live. If you give your body poor quality fuel, you will find your energy and health plummet. On the other hand, if you give your body healthy and high-quality fuel, you will increase your energy, well-being, and overall quality of life.

When on a standard Western diet, also frequently referred to as the Standard American Diet (SAD), people consume large quantities of carbs and highly processed additives. After we eat these carbs, whether it is ice cream and cookies or a bowl of pasta and French bread, these carbs are broken down into glucose by the body. This glucose is pure sugar, which is being fed to our cells as fuel.

When your body uses glucose as fuel, you get a temporary sugar-high, just like a child who gets a burst of energy after eating an ice cream cone. However, when this happens, insulin must be released by your pancreas in an attempt to manage the high blood sugar levels.

Sadly, this process which should go smoothly in healthy individuals frequently becomes impeded due to a variety of health conditions or old age. For instance, insulin resistance and reduced insulin sensitivity frequently can make it difficult for the insulin response to manage blood sugar, frequently leading to diabetes.

When insulin is unable to manage our blood sugar in a healthy way, then we experience two extremes. After all, for every action, there is an equal and opposite reaction. The first extreme you experience is the sugar high, and while this may give you a temporary surge of energy, it is frantic and unhealthy energy, one of which is only short-lasting.

After your short-lasting energy comes the sugar crash. Just as the sugar-high causes extreme jitters and energy, the sugar crash causes extreme fatigue, sleepiness, and headaches. Even people with a healthy insulin response experience this sugar high and crash, and it is only worsened as people age or develop insulin-related disorders.

While carbohydrates create glucose, a sugar, as a fuel source, the ketogenic diet greatly limits your carbohydrate intake. Because of this, instead of relying on quick sugar highs for energy, your body will rely on healthier and slower burning fuel sources. Fat and protein burn more slowly and without either a high or a crash, allowing your body to maintain a healthy and sustained energy level.

Not only will you have the longer burning fuel of fat and protein, but your body will also produce ketone bodies for fuel once you have adapted to the diet and reached the stage of ketosis. When this happens, the ketones will help fuel your body whenever you need an added boost of energy, ensuring that you have fewer energy crashes. No longer will you have to push through those dreaded afternoon slumps, Mondays will become easier, and you will find yourself drinking less caffeine. Between fat, protein, and ketones, you will be providing your body and cells with the best fuel sources they could hope for, allowing you to enjoy the all-day energy you have desired.

Mitochondrial Benefits

The mitochondrial cells, which are the cells that have the capability of using any of the fuel sources of energy, are incredibly powerful. The mitochondria within these cells are frequently referred to as the "powerhouse of the cell." The reason they are so powerful is that they produce ninety percent of the energy humans need to survive.

When we breathe the mitochondria, use a process known as oxidative phosphorylation to combine oxygen and the fuel we have eaten to create ATP energy. But, when there is a malfunction in the mitochondria, they are unable to fully produce the amount of ATP energy re requiring, resulting in damaged cells, tissues, and even organs.

These mitochondrial disorders can be inherited genetically or caused by various environmental factors. Thankfully, you can improve your mitochondrial and overall health by changing the fuel you feed your cells. By giving them higher quality fats, proteins, and ketones rather than low-quality glucose, you can impact the health of your entire body, as the mitochondrial cells make up such a large portion of your body.

Promising research has found that the ketogenic diet can increase the rate that mitochondrial cells synthesize energy, thereby reducing or preventing the energy deficiencies that go hand-in-hand with mitochondrial disorders. Not only that, but the ketogenic diet can also increase the number of mitochondrial cells found within the human body, increasing the energy even further.

Beautiful Healthy Skin and Hair

We all want to have beautiful skin and hair. But, as we age, they often lose their shine, become rough and course, and we may struggle with hair loss or skin rashes. When a person first begins the ketogenic diet, they may experience adverse side effects with their hair or skin, but this is due to the body's natural adjustment period. After you have been on the ketogenic diet for a few weeks or months, you should notice that your hair and skin begin to not only go back to normal but that they exceed their previous health.

This is largely due to overall body health allowing your skin and hair to become the best version of themselves, but it is also due to providing them better fuel. The cells within your hair and skin require fuel just like all your other cells, but frequently, these cells are not given enough healthy fat. This reduction in fat causes brittle hair that has lost its shine and dry itchy skin. But, if you provide these cells with healthy fats from avocados, olives, nuts, seeds, and fish, then you will find that they gain the luxurious health you have longed for.

Boost Eye Health

As we age, our eye health degenerates. Sometimes, this reveals itself simply with the vision becoming poorer and more blurry, but other times, it causes glaucoma to develop. This progressive condition causes damage to the cells that communicate visual information between the eyes and brain. What many people may not know is that if you have diabetes or a family history of diabetes, then you are at a higher risk of developing glaucoma. Thankfully, a study found that maintaining a ketogenic diet helps to protect these cells, allowing the eyes and brain to retain their communication connection and preserving eye health.

Improve Memory

As people grow older, the human brain begins to lose its ability to properly use glucose as an energy source. This is especially a problem since most people eat carb-heavy diets. The result? Due to the cells being unable to properly fuel themselves on glucose, they slowly starve, causing long-term chronic memory difficulties.

Thankfully, with the ketogenic diet, you can provide these cells with alternative fuel sources. Not only will they be provided with healthy fat and protein for fuel, but they will also have access to ketones. Ketones have been found to be the best source of fuel for human brain cells, meaning that you can improve your memory and general brain function as you age if you maintain the ketogenic diet.

Manage Blood Pressure

High blood pressure is a classic symptom of potential heart diseases and disorders that many people develop as they age. Doctors are consistently beginning to put more emphasis on the importance of maintaining blood pressure as research has proven that chronically high blood pressure can affect many other aspects of human health.

Often, we are told to lose weight to help manage blood pressure. Thankfully, the ketogenic diet can help with that, but it can also go beyond weight loss to improve your blood health. Many studies have found that when individuals follow a low-carb/high-fat (keto) diet, their blood pressure lowers to healthy levels, even without the use of medication. Many people have even been able to go off of their blood pressure medication and manage their blood and heart health completely with the ketogenic diet alone. Although, you should always manage your medication and diet with your doctor. Don't go off any medication without your doctor's help and approval.

Reduce Cancer Risk

While there is no one perfect way to treat cancer or reduce your risk of the disease, the ketogenic diet can help in many ways. Firstly, cancer is caused by free radicals and toxins in the body causing cellular harm and tumor growth. Yet, the ketogenic diet prioritizes foods that are antioxidants, which remove these harmful free radicals. Not only that, but while glucose forms free radicals during the process of being burned by fuel, ketones and fat do not. This means you can greatly reduce your risk of being cancer just by changing your cellular fuel source.

That is not all! Certain types of tumors can only grow and feed on glucose. This means that when you starve these tumor cells of the glucose they desire, they can no longer grow. They either stop growing or shrink altogether. While the rest of your cells can get the fuel they need from fat, protein, ketones, and the gluconeogenesis processes, the tumors will be forced to shrink.

Other studies have found that the ketogenic diet, when paired together with chemotherapy, is more effective in treating cancer. These studies found that by adding in the ketogenic diet in conjunction with chemotherapy, the therapy became more successful than it was on its own.

Remember, cancer prevention and treatment require many elements, and you can't simply eat a ketogenic diet and consider yourself healed. However, it is well documented that the ketogenic diet excels in helping those going through cancer treatment. By changing your diet and making other lifestyle and medication choices, you can greatly increase your health.

Reduce Inflammation, Joint Pain, and Treat Arthritis

Inflammation is an important part of the human immune system. This inflammation helps to fight infection, increase healing, ward off disease, and more. However, it is possible for inflammation levels to become chronically high, which can result in its own health problems. The dangers of high inflammation are especially seen in autoimmune diseases, such as rheumatoid arthritis.

Even if you don't have an autoimmune disease, you may still suffer from chronically high levels of inflammation. This inflammation will worsen joint pain and arthritis, interfere with sleep, progress anxiety and depression, and more.

But by reducing glucose intake and enjoying the ketogenic diet, which is full of anti-inflammatory foods, a person can directly lower their inflammation. Once inflammation lowers, you will find that you experience improvements in all areas of your health and life, including a decrease in joint and arthritis pain.

Treat Diabetes and Blood Sugar

The glucose found within high-carb foods causes high blood sugar and insulin response to help manage this glucose. But, if a person has insulin resistance or diabetes, this mechanism for the body will not work properly, leading to chronically high blood sugar and a series of other health issues. Thankfully, there is much you can do to fix this through diet. Some people may require medication, which is something you can only have answered by your doctor, but if you add the ketogenic diet into your life, you can improve your overall health, manage your blood sugar, and possibly even reduce any blood pressure medication you might be on.

When on the standard Western diet, a person's blood sugar is practically on a roller coaster ride, going up and down throughout the day as they get blood sugar highs and lows from glucose. But on the ketogenic diet, you ride on a reliable and trustworthy ship rather than a roller coaster. This is because fat, protein, and ketones all offer more sustained and long-term energy that doesn't cause spikes or lows.

Over time, as your blood sugar remains stable due to the reduction in glucose and a diet of healthier food sources, a person's insulin response will begin to heal and repair itself, often causing insulin resistance to reverse itself. After a period of months of the ketogenic diet, many people can stop or reduce their blood sugar medication, but this can only be done under a doctor's close guidance.

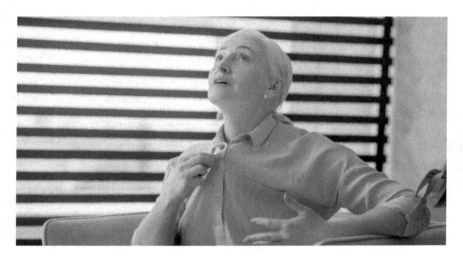

Help for Pre and Post Menopause

The symptoms of menopause can come at different ages for different women and the symptoms can vary. But, the universal truth is that no matter your age or symptoms, menopause can be a challenge. This is because not only is menopause a new way of life, but the change in hormones can cause weight gain, mood swings, insomnia, hot flashes, changes in libido, and more.

These side effects are caused by changes in the hormones testosterone and estrogen. Thankfully, the ketogenic diet can help you to balance these hormones so that your symptoms subside, all thanks to increasing healthy fats and reducing glucose in your diet. The top six ways you will experience improvement with the ketogenic diet for menopause-related symptoms include:

1. Hormonal balance
2. Insulin control
3. Body temperature regulation
4. Weight management
5. Improved sleep
6. Increased energy levels

Weight Loss

Weight loss is not an easy or one-size-fits-all matter. Thankfully, while there may not be a single solution to the weight problems of the entire planet, studies have shown that the ketogenic diet is one of the most effective options we have. This is because when we no longer are constantly putting more glucose in our bodies, we begin to burn fat and ketones instead. Because our body is burning this ingested fat and ketones, it will also burn more body fat, allowing you to naturally lose weight.

But, that is not all! Fat and protein are much more satisfying than carbohydrates. This means that you can eat fewer calories than you would if you were eating carbohydrates, but still feel more full and satisfied for longer. This process will naturally allow you to go longer without eating, as you simply won't be hungry, resulting in further weight loss.

You can even go a step further in boosting your weight loss by implementing healthy short-term intermittent fasting, which we will cover in a later chapter.

Metabolic Syndrome and Cholesterolemia

The layperson may be unaware of what metabolic syndrome is, but, it is a series of problems that affect the world at large. More specifically, it is a collection of symptoms that are linked to heart disease and type II diabetes. There are many possible signs and symptoms, but some of the most common is high blood sugar, raised blood pressure, increased blood triglyceride levels, low (good) HDL cholesterol levels, and increased waist size.

As you know from our previous points, the ketogenic diet can help each and every one of these points. Multiple studies have compared a variety of exercises and diets in the treatment of metabolic syndrome, and these studies have found that the ketogenic diet excels above all the other options.

Osteoporosis

Osteoporosis is a concern we all must think about as we age. It is all too common for people to begin breaking bones and receiving joint replacements as they grow older. But, there are ways you can decrease your risk of osteoporosis and increase your overall bone health.

Many people only think that calcium is important for bone health, and therefore, they suggest drinking more milk. But, milk is high in glucose. While other dairies may be allowed on the ketogenic diet, milk is not beneficial. So, where does that leave you with osteoporosis? Surprisingly to many people, this is actually better for your bone health. This is because studies have found that humans largely are unable to absorb the calcium found within milk and that it rarely aides in bone health. Instead, you would do much better in gaining calcium from non-dairy sources, such as:

- Sardines (bone-in)
- Nuts
- Cabbage
- Kale
- Okra
- Broccoli
- Collard Greens

But, more than calcium, you should focus on increasing your vitamin D intake. This is because humans are unable to utilize calcium without first having enough vitamin D. Sadly, over half of the population in the Western world has vitamin D deficiencies, which is why the number of people with osteoporosis is so high. Thankfully, there are several ways you can improve your vitamin D intake, and therefore, your bone health. First, by spending thirty minutes outside in the sun a day, you can greatly increase your vitamin D levels, but you can also get it in the food you eat. Try eating more:

- Fatty Fish
- Eggs
- Shrimp
- Oysters
- Mushrooms
- Beef Liver

It's important to remember that you shouldn't simply eat any keto-friendly food. You need to focus on eating a balanced diet that incorporates a range of nutrients, like the ones mentioned here. If you include a variety of keto-friendly vegetables, nuts, seeds, fats, and protein sources, you will find that your health begins to greatly improve.

Chapter 5: How to Begin the Ketogenic Diet

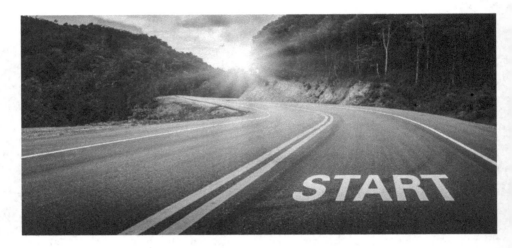

Before ever beginning the ketogenic diet, there are two things you need to do:

1. Research and understand the subject – Congratulations, by reading this book, you are well on your way to completing this step!
2. Have a checkup and talk with your doctor.

Once you have an understanding of the keto process, you need to discuss the diet with your doctor and how your specific health might affect the diet. For instance, if you have high cholesterol, hormonal imbalances, diabetes, or one of any number of other conditions, your doctor can discuss the effects with you. Your doctor should discuss any potential risks, how to prevent dangers, and any potential benefits. For instance, if you have high cholesterol, your doctor might discuss with you how you should prioritize unsaturated fats such as avocado and olive oil instead of saturated fats from meat and dairy.

Your doctor will also want to keep an eye on any medication you are on, in case it needs to be adjusted after being on the ketogenic diet for a time. While some people might have to stay on their medications, others might find so much improvement that they can reduce their dosage or completely go off of their medication. But, this can only be done under close watch by your doctor.

Lastly, you should ask your doctor to run some basic tests that they can use for a baseline in the future. For instance, you might ask them to check your cholesterol, blood pressure, weight, and general vitamin and mineral blood tests. By having these tests as a baseline, your doctor can let you know how your overall keto progress is going.

After discussing the plan thoroughly with your doctor, you should set up a schedule to check back with them on your keto progress. Your doctor will know how long you should wait between visits. If you are rather healthy, you may not need to see them for a few months, then you can do a post-keto checkup. But, if you have a chronic illness or disease, you might want to see them once a month for a few months, just until both you and your doctor can see proven results.

The Keto Flu

When you first begin the ketogenic diet, it is common to go into what is known as the "keto flu." This is the hardest part of the ketogenic diet, as it is when your body is going through the transition of relying on glucose to switching to a protein, fat, and ketone fuel source. There are different stages of the keto flu, and thankfully, they are not all difficult.

The most difficult stage of the keto flu is the first few days, or up to a week, that you are on the diet. During this stage, your body is burning off any glucose stored within your body. Your cells can't begin to produce ketones until it burns off this glucose. For people with healthy insulin responses, this should only take between two to three days depending on activity level and pre-keto diet. But, for people with insulin resistance or diabetes, it can take up to a week.

You will lose the most weight during the first week, but not due to fat loss. While a small percentage of this weight loss might be fat, it will mostly be water weight. Water molecules naturally attach to glucose in the body, and when this glucose is burned off, your body dumps the excess water, resulting in rapid weight loss. This rapid water loss can lead to both dehydration and electrolyte deficiencies, so it is important to remember to drink plenty of fluids and consume more electrolytes in your food. Most often, adverse effects like headaches can be caused not only due to the transition between pre-keto to keto but due to dehydration and electrolyte deficiencies. If you take care to prevent these two side effects with proper care, you will find that you feel much better.

Once the body has begun to produce ketones, you will begin to feel better. However, there are three types of ketones. When you first begin the ketogenic diet, you will only be producing one type of ketone. After two to three weeks on the ketogenic diet, you will go into a "deep ketosis" in which your body begins to produce the more effective forms of ketones. After you go into deep ketosis, you will find your energy levels going up, and you start to receive more health benefits. The exact time period differs for everyone, but you should enter deep ketosis by the end of your first full month on keto.

Let's look at some possible adverse effects people might experience, and how you can overcome them.

Bad Breath:
The bad breath you experience on the ketogenic diet usually occurs somewhere between the end of week one and the beginning of week four. As there are three different types of ketones, this symptom occurs when the first type (acetone) is dumped from the body when it is no longer needed. Since acetone is not as effective as the other two ketones (acetoacetate and beta-hydroxybutyrate) when you enter deep ketosis and begin to produce the more effective ketones, your body will get rid of the unneeded acetone through your breath and urine. This can give off a weird smell, but thankfully, only lasts a few days or up to one week. All you can do to help with this is to mask it by using breath mints, but it won't last long.

Dry Mouth:
Dry mouth comes to dehydration. As we mentioned previously, while the keto flu can cause mild side effects while your body is adjusting such as aches, insomnia, and nausea, they shouldn't be overly severe. If you find that your keto flu feels particularly strong, then it might be dehydration and electrolyte deficiencies. One way you might be able to tell if this is the problem is if you are having a dry mouth. If this happens, simply make sure you are drinking plenty of water and consuming your doctor's recommended daily dose of electrolytes.
In general, it is recommended that humans drink at least half their body's weight in ounces daily. This means that if you weigh one-hundred and fifty pounds, then you should drink at least seventy-five fluid ounces of water daily. You can drink more than this, but if you drink more, keep in mind that you will need a higher dose of electrolytes.

Never drink more than one liter within the span of an hour, no matter how thirsty you feel or how dry your mouth is. Drinking more than this rapidly will damage your liver. If you can't get rid of the dry mouth, try sucking on some sugar-free mints that are sweetened with sugar alcohols.

Digestive Upset:
The ketogenic diet may cause digestive upset in people when they first start. Some people don't have any problems, whereas others will have one of two extremes: constipation or diarrhea. While unpleasant, thankfully, both of these are easy to fix on the ketogenic diet.

Constipation is usually a sign of two possible keto mistakes. First, either the person is dehydrated. Or, second, the person isn't eating enough fiber. If a person isn't eating enough low-carb high-fiber vegetables, it can really mess up their digestion, so make sure you eat plenty of keto-friendly veggies! If you are still having problems, try drinking some bulletproof coffee with MCT oil. Between the magnesium in the coffee and the medium-chain triglycerides in the fat, you should have no problems in no time.

It likely means that you are not eating enough fiber, which is needed to bulk up your stools, or that you are eating too much MCT oil. Since MCT oil is processed by the body more quickly than long-chain fatty acids, it can cause a person to experience diarrhea. If you experience this, back off on the MCT oil and choose other fats such as avocado, olive, nuts, and seeds instead.

Insomnia:
Insomnia may be caused due to a change in your diet. Insomnia does not have a single quick fix, but there are a few things that can help. First, try not to eat within three hours of bedtime, as fats are high caloric, and the energy from them may leave you restless.

Try to stick with a nightly routine that is peaceful, practice meditation or mindfulness before bed, lower overall life stress, and try practicing light exercise early during the morning or afternoon.

Even if you are not experiencing insomnia, try to include mindfulness, meditation, and yoga. While the ketogenic diet is amazing and powerful, it is important to remember if you want improvements in your whole life, then you need to take a whole-life approach. By making changes to not only what you eat but when you eat, how you sleep, and including healthier lifestyle activities during the day, then you will reap all the benefits you have hoped for. Your doctor will be happy, as well, since these practices have proven to calm the mind, lower blood pressure, and lead to other positive physical and mental changes.

But, just to make these positive changes doesn't mean you have to completely change your schedule. You don't have to start a class or start waking up two hours earlier in the morning. All you have to do is set aside fifteen minutes a day to practice mindfulness in a quiet room, or find thirty minutes when you can incorporate yoga. There are plenty of resources available, no class needed!

Alkaline Keto Foods

There is still only a limited number of studies showing the effects of acidic and alkaline food on human health. However, proponents of the alkaline diet have long believed that by incorporating more alkaline foods to balance out the acidic foods we eat that we could benefit our health.

In general, many people on the ketogenic diet do not consider whether the given food is alkaline or not. But, it is worth noting that there are many believers in the alkaline diet, and if you choose to combine the ketogenic diet and alkaline properties, then you can reap the rewards.

It is believed that when a person eats a highly acidic diet, it throws off the body's natural pH balance, leading to heart disease, cancer, osteoporosis, diabetes, and other conditions. This is why I recommend drinking alkaline water, instead of tap water.

The animal proteins found on the ketogenic diet are known to be acid-forming foods, but you can decrease any associated risk from eating these meats by pairing them with other more alkaline ingredients. Foods are not either okay or not okay based on whether they are alkaline or not. It is all about gaining balance over the two.

When you digest food, it is broken down into metabolic waste, which can then be classified as either acidic, neutral, or alkaline. Anything with a pH under seven is acidic, with a perfect seven being neutral, and over seven being alkaline. While it has yet to be proven, it is believed that when you eat foods at a variety of points on this scale, it will affect your body's own pH. For instance, if you eat a lot of acidic food, your body's pH will lower. Whereas, if you eat a lot of alkaline food, your pH will rise. But, if you balance both acidic and alkaline foods as part of your daily diet, you can maintain a healthy and balanced pH.

Foods that are known to create an acidic response include meat, eggs, fish, dairy, grains, and alcohol. Then, foods that create an alkaline response include vegetables, fruits, nuts, seeds, and legumes.

As you can see, the ketogenic diet contains a fair number of foods from both categories, while also not allowing those from others. For example, you avoid grains and alcohol from the acidic category, but also avoid legumes and many fruits from the alkaline portion. This means that with the ketogenic diet, you can naturally gain a balance over your pH.

While the science behind the alkaline diet has not yet been proven, thankfully, there is no harm in implementing and potentially benefiting from it! After all, all you have to do to benefit from it is include more healthy alkaline foods. This means you can increase the number of low-carb vegetables you eat daily, improving your overall health. Even though the pH diet may not be proven, the health benefits of low-carb vegetables have been proven, and any doctor would encourage you to eat more.

Eat healthy whole foods, keep carbs to a minimum, and choose the healthiest fat options. You will not regret making the change to go keto.

Chapter 6: Best Foods to Choose for Success

In this chapter, we will focus on the foods you should focus on in the ketogenic diet. We previously discussed the best fats to choose, which you should enjoy liberally within your specific caloric intake needs. This means you can enjoy a delicious bacon omelet fried in butter for breakfast, a salmon with avocado and roasted vegetables at lunch, and maybe a bulletproof coffee complete with MCT oil and grass-fed butter at some point during your day. But, while fats make up a large and important part of the ketogenic diet, there are other many aspects you need to focus on, as well. Since we have previously discussed the fats involved, in this chapter, we will focus on other food options you have to choose from.

Choose Organic:
Organic food contains fewer pesticides, it's fresher, tastes better, and is better for the environment. Organic animal-based products have not been treated with antibiotics or hormones, which can cause antibiotic-resistant bacteria and diseases to form. Lastly, whether plant or animal, organic products are higher in nutrients.

How your food is grown, raised, and treated impacts how it affects your body and mind. This is plain to see in every food choice you make. For instance, nobody will argue that the fat from avocados and olives is healthier for you than the harmful trans fats found in highly processed foods. While we can't always buy the highest quality ingredients, due to their price, when able, it is wise to make the best food choices you can. For instance, you may not be able to buy all your produce organic, but you might be able to afford to buy specific ingredients that are on the "dirty dozen" list (such as strawberries) organic. By doing this, you can make the best choices for your health while also saving money.

Grass-Fed Meat:
As we previously discussed in the chapter about fat, there is a big difference in the quality of grass-fed dairy products and grain-fed. This is not only true of the dairy produced from animals, but also the meat itself. Grass-fed meat is always superior, no matter the animal source. But, once a case in which you can especially see superiority, is when it comes to beef. This is because

beef is especially affected by the different food sources: grass-fed beef containing an amazingly high level of nutrition.

Grass-fed beef may cost more, but it is worth buying as frequently as possible. Even if you can only buy grass-fed beef once a week, the nutritional benefits would be worth it. When possible, try to buy grass-fed beef liver, as it is the most nutritionally dense portion of the meat. Even if you don't usually like organ meats; if the liver is chopped up and mixed with ground beef, you will never notice that it is there.

When buying your grass-fed beef, look for a stamp certifying it by the American Grass-fed Association (AGA) to ensure that it is from a trustworthy source. The AGA makes sure that all products certified were always fed with grass, never grains, and that they were never given either hormones or antibiotics.

Some benefits of grass-fed beef include:

- Lower in calories
- Increased number of healthy fats
- Contains fewer bacteria
- Supports healthy blood sugar levels
- Contains important vitamins and minerals
- Fights cancer and heart disease

Sweetener Choices:

There are three main sweetener choices you will enjoy on the ketogenic diet, which are stevia, erythritol, and monk fruit. We will go over these three options here.

Erythritol is a sugar-free natural sweetener. While this sweetener is classified as a sugar alcohol, it does not contain either glucose or alcohol. Instead, it gets its name from being a type of fermented sweetener naturally found within the fruit that is not digested by the body. In the same way that fiber isn't digested and is then expelled from the body, so too is erythritol.

Erythritol has a light taste that goes well in most baked goods, has no effect on blood sugar, and is easy on the stomach in moderate servings. Although, large servings might cause some slight stomach upset.

Similar to erythritol is xylitol, which is another form of sugar alcohol. While they are similar, xylitol more frequently causes stomach upset. While you can enjoy both forms of sugar alcohol on the ketogenic diet, erythritol is generally thought to be superior.

Monk fruit sweetener has become more popular in recent years, as it is another natural sugar-free sweetener. While most fruits contain high levels of glucose and fructose, the sweetener found within the monk fruit is different. This melon-like fruit is two-hundred times sweeter than cane sugar, yet it contains no calories. This sweetness is not due to any type of actual sweetener, but due to a natural and healthy compound that only tastes "sweet", known as mogrosides. Monk fruit is free of carbs, doesn't affect insulin, and is perfectly safe.

Stevia leaf is similar in some ways to monk fruit. Like monk fruit, stevia is a natural plant that tastes sweet, yet contains no actual sweetener. Stevia leaf has been found to be about one-hundred and fifty times as sweet as cane sugar but has no effect on blood sugar or insulin. Frequently, stevia and erythritol will be combined together and sold as low-carb baking blends or other low-calorie foods. You can often find stevia sold as a crystallized powder or as a liquid tincture, but you can also grow this herb in your own backyard.

Alkaline Water:
Alkaline water is different from tap water, as its pH level is much less acidic. While the pH scale ranges from zero to fourteen from acidic to alkaline, the pH scale of alkaline water has been increased. In general, tap water will have a pH scale of seven, making it moderately acidic. On the other hand, alkaline water has a pH scale of eight or nine, making it less acidic and supposedly giving its health benefits.

Alkaline water contains minerals that help to make it less acidic and negative oxidation-reduction potential (ORP), which have the ability to act as an antioxidant.

Don't Go Overboard on Protein:
Protein is an important and vital macronutrient, which you must ensure you eat enough of. If you do not eat enough protein, then your muscles will not be able to maintain their mass, and your cells will be deprived of an important nutrient source. Remember, while the human body does not need to eat carbohydrates, it does need to eat protein and fats.

But, while you certainly need to make sure you are eating your daily requirements of protein, you don't need to go overboard, either. If you eat more protein than you require, all you are doing is increasing your caloric intake and possibly even increase your intake of moderate value fats rather than high-quality fats.

In order to make sure you don't go overboard on your protein intake, you should use a keto macro ratio calculator to determine your specific protein needs. While the calculator can give you a specific number, usually, a healthy protein intake range is 0.7 to 0.9 grams of protein for every pound of body weight.

Chapter 7: Increasing the Benefits with Intermittent Fasting

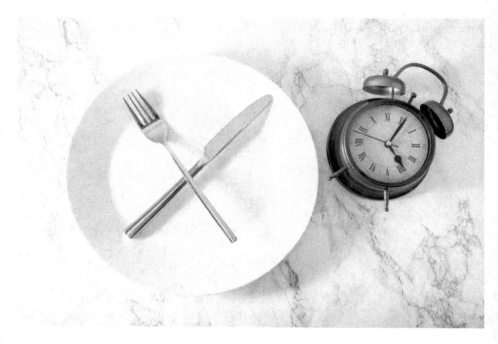

I'm sure you've heard, and maybe even repeated, phrases such as "breakfast is the most important meal of the day," and "if you skip a meal, your metabolism will slow down." Yet, these phrases are based largely on misinformation. Studies have long shown that there are many health benefits to practicing short-term fasting, known as intermittent fasting. This is good news, as intermittent fasting is made easy and accessible on the ketogenic diet.

Generally, intermittent fasting is practiced no longer than twenty-four hours, although this is only for people who are more advanced in their fasting journey. Longer fasting periods are never needed, many people never fast for longer than twelve or sixteen hours. This may seem like a long time, but it really is not. Many people might already practice twelve-hour intermittent fasting without trying, as we all fast overnight while we are asleep. This means that if you finish dinner at seven in the evening and eat breakfast at seven in the morning, you have completed a twelve-hour fast.

On the ketogenic diet, it becomes easier to practice intermittent fasting than with the standard western diet, as you are no longer experiencing blood sugar highs and crashes from glucose. Instead, you are being sustained on protein, fat, and ketones, which will keep you full and sustained for longer periods. You don't force yourself to go longer periods between meals, you simply wait to eat when you are hungry, which over time, will lengthen into slightly longer periods. When many people begin the ketogenic diet, they may eat four small meals a day as their body adjusts. Yet, over time, as they adjust to the change in fuel sources, they will be able to find themselves naturally satisfied and able to eat two or three large meals a day instead.

The way everyone adjusts to the ketogenic diet and intermittent fasting is different, there is no reason to push yourself to do it in one specific way. Allow your body to do what it needs, listen to its signals, eat when you feel hungry, and don't eat when you aren't hungry. Many people may eat even if they aren't hungry due to being bored or in the habit of eating regularly, but this will only impede your weight loss goals.

If you don't want to practice intermittent fasting, that is okay. You don't have to practice it right away or ever, or you might decide to change your mind in the future. It doesn't matter. You can choose what is best for your body and situation. Intermittent fasting, while helpful in increasing health and weight loss, isn't a necessary part of the ketogenic diet. Many people choose to first adjust to the ketogenic diet before deciding whether or not to take up intermittent fasting, as it is easiest to make one change at a time.

Before we discuss how you can practice intermittent fasting, let's look at some of the benefits beyond weight loss.

HGH Hormone:
The human growth hormone is produced within the pituitary gland, and it's one of our most vital hormones. It is at its highest level during periods of growth and decreases in individuals as we age. While this hormone has many important roles, some of the more common include maintaining brain health, muscle mass, bone density, tissue health, and more.

With these important roles of the HGH hormone, it is easy to see why a decrease in the hormone causes problems. As we age, this decrease causes us to lose muscle mass. We develop osteoporosis. Our tissues become stretched, thin, and easily damaged. Thankfully, we can also increase our HGH hormone naturally through our diets. It is well established that fasting increases our HGH production. This means that if you practice intermittent fasting a couple of times a week, or even daily, you can boost your human growth hormone level up to five times its baseline level.

Reduce Oxidative Stress:

Our aging is greatly increased by oxidative stress done by free radicals. As we have discussed, the ketogenic diet is a great way to reduce the number of free radicals in your body and the damage they can achieve. However, that does not mean there isn't more progress to be made. The ketogenic diet is a great start, and by implementing intermittent fasting, you can take this a step further and receive even more benefits. As intermittent fasting reduces oxidative stress, you can slow the rate of cellular decay, reduce the risk of disease, and age more gracefully.

Increase Heart Health:

The leading cause of death worldwide is heart disease, causing over thirty-one percent of deaths annually. Despite increasing awareness by medical professionals, there is still much that the layperson does not understand about their heart health. We still make many mistakes. Thankfully, we can also make choices to improve our heart health. The ketogenic diet and intermittent fasting have both been found to be wonderful choices to promote further heart health and decrease the risk of cardiac-related events.

There have been multiple studies on the subject, with one study finding that when people practiced intermittent fasting daily for two months, they were able to reduce their bad cholesterol by twenty-five percent. Not only that, but they also reduced their blood triglyceride level by thirty-two percent.

Boost Cellular Health:

The human body goes through a process known as autophagy. During this process, our old damaged cells are replaced with young and healthy cells, allowing us to flourish. Think about it this way: when your skin is dry and itchy, you will clear away the dead skin cells that are in the way before you hydrate the young and healthy cells. By replacing the old with the new, you allow your body to become the best version of itself.

Autophagy is the body's natural process of doing this. It is a vital process that helps to prevent disease and slow down aging. Scientists have long sought a way to replicate the autophagy process through medication to help in the treatment of diseases. But, while there is not yet a medication that can stimulate this response, intermittent fasting can trigger the autophagy response.

Increase Brain Health:

There are many diseases and disorders that affect the brain. Some of these commonly first occur at birth or during early adulthood, such as epilepsy, depression, or bipolar disorder. On the other hand, there are many disorders that, by and large, affect people as they age, such as Alzheimer's disease. While these disorders may have many different causes and possible treatments, there is one thing that will clearly help all of them: healthier brain cells. Intermittent fasting is able to help with this, as studies show that the practice of fasting increases brain cell growth and regeneration. By increasing this, we are able to boost overall brain performance as well as memory, focus, and mood. Whether you are hoping to simply increase your memory and daily brain function or hope to lower your risk of developing dementia in the future, you will be happy to know that regular intermittent fasting can help.

These benefits are only the tip of the iceberg! Whether you choose to start intermittent fasting slowly by pushing back your mealtime an hour or decide to jump right in with a twelve, fourteen, or even sixteen-hour fast, you will find benefit. While there are a few guidelines to follow while fasting, there is not one specific method of fasting that you have to stick with. Once you understand the methods, you can then apply them in whatever way feels more natural. But, to do this, you need to understand what to do and not to do, so make sure you understand the dos and don'ts before you switch things up.

When you are adjusted to fasting, you should go through your fasting period sustained and full, without feeling the need to snack. This is because the fuels you will be eating are long-burning fuels, unlike glucose. While glucose can give you rapid sugar highs and crashes, the fuels on the ketogenic diet will not. But, when you first begin the ketogenic diet, you will find yourself still getting hungry more frequently, as your body is not yet adjusted to the change in fuel sources and has not learned how to fully adjust to producing ketones. It usually takes four to six weeks to fully adjust. Because of this, many people will put off intermittent fasting until this period, because you don't want to fast when you are hungry. Fasting when hungry is just setting yourself up for failure when instead you want to give yourself every opportunity to succeed.

Whenever you eat, you enter what is known as the fed state. This phase is when your body is working on digesting food, and it lasts three to five hours. During this time, your body is unlikely to burn any of your body fat, as all of its work is going to be digesting and burning what you have just eaten.

After this three to five-hour period, you enter the post-absorptive state. This phase begins when you finish digesting food, but are still somewhat satisfied. Your insulin levels will be lower, and you will find you are more likely to burn body fat and excess calories during this time. This state starts between three and five hours after eating, and it can last between eight to twelve hours. Most individuals don't go past the post-absorptive state in their daily lives in modern society, as we have normalized regular meal times.

After eight to twelve hours, a person exits the post-absorptive state and enters the fasted state. During this state is when you receive the most benefits from intermittent fasting. You not only burn the most fat and lose the most weight in this state, but when you are in the fasted state is when you also reap all the cellular and neurological benefits. For this reason, many people try to work up to sixteen-hour fasts, so that they can get at least a few hours in the fasted state whenever they practice intermittent fasting.

Fasting used to be a normal and healthy part of everyday human life. Actually, in some cultures, it is still a normal daily aspect of life. However, in today's modern Western society, we are conditioned to believe that we need to eat at least three large meals a day. Some people even decide to spread this out further, eating up to six small meals a day instead! This may be necessary for people with specific medical conditions, but in general, this is not beneficial for human health. Our digestion shouldn't always be in the "on" position like a car engine always running. The phases of digestion and fasting are important aspects of human biology, and by putting these phases to use, we can experience better health and weight loss.

When beginning intermittent fasting, most people will begin with short fasting windows, which they slowly extend over time. For instance, if you usually eat breakfast at six and lunch at noon, you might try pushing lunch back two hours later in the day than usual. But, don't force yourself. If you try to force yourself through fasting while hungry, not only will you be miserable, but you will likely overeat later on when you break your fast. To help yourself fast for longer periods while staying full and satisfied, start out with eating a large and satisfying meal full of healthy proteins and fats before beginning your fast.

While there are many schedule types for intermittent fasting, there are a few that are particularly ideal for women fifty and over. In this chapter, we will go over my favorite three methods.

Twelve-Twelve Fast:

The twelve-twelve fast is ideal for the beginner, as most of us already go twelve hours without eating overnight as we sleep. However, it is also important to remember that the post-absorptive stage lasts between hours eight and twelve after eating, meaning you might not receive the full range of benefits as you would with longer fasting windows. While the shorter fasting window may not be as effective, don't let that push you toward trying longer fasting windows before you are ready. By starting out with a manageable twelve-hour fasting window, you can give yourself time to adjust and succeed, and later on, you can slowly lengthen your fasting window to increase the benefits.

When practicing the twelve-hour fast, you will want to schedule it so that a majority of it takes place while you sleep, allowing you to eat breakfast in the morning before you leave for work.

Sixteen-Eight Fast:
One of the most common fasting options is the sixteen-eight fast, also known as the Leangains diet. This fasting period is wonderful because, with a sixteen-hour fasting window, a person can benefit from all the health and weight loss benefits of the fasting phase, but without it being overly intense. Sure, fasting for sixteen hours may seem intense at first. But, after you have been on the ketogenic diet for a time and your body adjusts to fueling off of sustained fat, protein, and ketones, then you will find that you can easily maintain this length of fast. Don't feel like you have to jump right into the sixteen-eight fast. You can start with a twelve-twelve fast and slowly lengthen the fasting window by thirty to sixty minutes at a time until you fully adjust.

If you want, you may choose to further customize this fasting option. Instead of starting out with a twelve-twelve fasting window and lengthening it to a sixteen-eight window, you may find that another option works better for you. For instance, some women find that fourteen-hour fast works are better for them than sixteen, so they stick with that without ever attempting to lengthen the fast further. After all, if it works, why try to change it? You can find what naturally works for you.

Twice Weekly Fast:
While some people prefer to have a standard fasting window they stick with daily, others prefer to fast on specific days of the week. When fasting this way, you can fast for as long or as short as you would like, up to twenty-four hours, that is. When a person completes a twice-weekly twenty-four hour fast, women will consume up to five-hundred calories on their fasting days, to

help ensure they meet their minimal required nutrition. These calories should originate from healthy foods and prioritize fats, proteins, and micronutrients.

If you choose to do a twice-weekly twenty-four hour fast, you shouldn't do two days back-to-back. This fasting schedule is set up so that you have eating days between fasting days so that you can fully nourish your body. Always have at least one day between your fasting days, but ideally two to three days. Don't feel as if you have to go a full twenty-four hours fasting, as this is the extreme end of intermittent fasting. If you want to do a twice-weekly fast at eighteen or twenty hours instead of twenty-four, that is perfectly okay! Make the schedule work best for your needs.

Chapter 8: 21-Day Meal Plan

In this chapter, you will be receiving a three-week menu plan to help you excel on the ketogenic diet. While you can certainly enjoy this menu plan as-is, you should also feel free to switch things up with your favorite healthy keto-friendly ingredients and meals, if you wish.

Day 1:

Breakfast:
Cheesy Sausage and Egg Bites

Lunch:
Chicken salad with artichoke hearts, avocado, and tomatoes served over a bed of spinach

Dinner:
Chicken BLT Lettuce Wraps

Snack/Dessert:
Toll House-Style Chocolate Chip Cookies

Day 2:

Breakfast:
Chia pudding made with coconut milk, raspberries, and lemon

Lunch:
Sliced turkey breast with Creamy Broccoli Salad

Dinner:
Shrimp scampi with zucchini noodles

Snack/Dessert:
Italian Cream Cake

Day 3:

Breakfast:
Low-carb cloud bread with poached eggs, ham, Hollandaise sauce, and asparagus spears

Lunch:
Salad with salmon, almonds, blueberries, and avocado dressing

Dinner:
Beef stroganoff with zucchini or spaghetti squash noodles

Snack/Dessert:
Blueberry Crumble Bars

Day 4:

Breakfast:
Eggs fried in butter with mushrooms and tomatoes

Lunch:
Roasted broccoli with sardines

Dinner:
Bok choy and cabbage stir-fry with shrimp

Snack/Dessert:
Key Lime Curd Bars

Day 5:

Breakfast:
Vegetable quiche with low-carb crust

Lunch:
Creamy Parmesan Noodles

Dinner:
Zucchini noodle lasagna with meat sauce

Snack/Dessert:
Bacon Deviled Eggs

Day 6:

Breakfast:
Bullet-proof coffee with MCT oil, collagen, and ketone powder

Lunch:
Teriyaki tofu with stir-fry

Dinner:
Spaghetti squash with meatballs and marinara

Snack/Dessert:
Strawberry Shortcake

Day 7:

Breakfast:
Cream Cheese Pancakes

Lunch:
Stuffed bell peppers with mushrooms, turkey, and tomato

Dinner:
Cloud bread sandwich with turkey, bacon, avocado, and tomato

Snack/Dessert:
Thin Mint Cookies

Day 8:

Breakfast:
Roasted egg stuffed avocado with cheese

Lunch:
Salmon cakes with sauteed spinach and tartar sauce

Dinner:
Shrimp scampi with zucchini noodles

Snack/Dessert:
Pumpkin Pie Cheesecake Bars

Day 9:

Breakfast:
Bacon and bell pepper omelet

Lunch:
Cloud bread sandwich with roasted mushrooms, bell peppers, and low-carb cauliflower hummus

Dinner:
Bok choy and cabbage stir-fry with shrimp

Snack/Dessert:
Key Lime Curd Bars

Day 10:

Breakfast:
Keto Pancake breakfast sandwich with egg, cheese, and bacon

Lunch:
Pan-fried cauliflower with bacon, cheese, and chicken

Dinner:
Eggplant Lasagna with beef sauce and cheese

Snack/Dessert:
Toll House-Style Chocolate Chip Cookies

Day 11:

Breakfast:
Vegetable frittata

Lunch:
Chicken salad with artichoke hearts, avocado, and tomatoes served over a bed of spinach

Dinner:
Cheeseburger Wraps

Snack/Dessert:
Better-Than-Reese's Almond Butter Cups

Day 12:

Breakfast:
Bulletproof coffee with MCT oil, collagen, and ketone powder

Lunch:
Parmesan Garlic Roasted Green Beans

Dinner:
Lamb chops with roasted squash and Brussels sprouts

Snack/Dessert:
Dill Pickle Snack Rolls

Day 13:

Breakfast:
Eggs fried in butter with mushrooms and tomatoes

Lunch:
Oven-roasted sardines with capers and herb seasoning served with roasted green beans

Dinner:
Pot roast with roasted radishes

Snack/Dessert:
Pumpkin Pie Cheesecake Bars

Day 14:

Breakfast:
Chia seed pudding with soy milk and chocolate

Lunch:
Chicken BLT Lettuce Wraps

Dinner:
Zucchini noodle lasagna with meat sauce

Snack/Dessert:
Bacon Deviled Eggs

Day 15:

Breakfast:
Cream Cheese Pancakes

Lunch:
Roasted broccoli with sardines

Dinner:
Stuffed bell peppers with mushrooms, turkey, and tomato

Snack/Dessert:
Thin Mint Cookies

Day 16:

Breakfast:
Fried eggs and cauliflower hash browns

Lunch:
Sliced turkey breast with Creamy Broccoli Salad

Dinner:

Snack/Dessert:
Toll House-Style Chocolate Chip Cookies

Day 17:

Breakfast:
Vegetable frittata

Lunch:
Salad with salmon, almonds, blueberries, and avocado dressing

Dinner:
Beef stroganoff with zucchini or spaghetti squash noodles

Snack/Dessert:
Italian Cream Cake

Day 18:

Breakfast:
Keto Pancake breakfast sandwich with egg, cheese, and bacon

Lunch:
Creamy Parmesan Noodles

Dinner:
Spaghetti squash with meatballs and marinara

Snack/Dessert:
Dill Pickle Snack Rolls

Day 19:

Breakfast:
Roasted egg stuffed avocado with cheese

Lunch:
Cloud bread sandwich with turkey, bacon, avocado, and tomato

Dinner:
Teriyaki tofu with stir-fry

Snack/Dessert:
Strawberry Shortcake

Day 20:

Breakfast:
Fried eggs and cauliflower hash browns

Lunch:
Oven-roasted sardines with capers and herb seasoning served with roasted green beans

Dinner:
Cheeseburger Wraps

Snack/Dessert:
Mascarpone Brownies

Day 21:

Breakfast:
Cheesy Sausage and Egg Bites

Lunch:
Parmesan Garlic Roasted Green Beans

Dinner:
Pot roast with roasted radishes

Snack/Dessert:
No-Bake Cheesecake

Chapter 9: Recipes

Cheesy Sausage and Egg Bites

These bites are the perfect breakfast, as you can just grab a few out of the fridge and go! Eat them either warm or cold, either way, you will find that they are delicious.

The Details:
The Number of Servings: 5
The Time Needed to Prepare: 20 minutes
The Time Required to Cook: 20 minutes
The Total Preparation/Cook Time: 40 minutes
Number of Calories in Individual Servings: 413
Protein Grams: 23
Fat Grams: 33
Total Carbohydrates Grams: 4
Net Carbohydrates Grams: 3.5

The Ingredients:
Cheddar cheese, shredded – 1 cup
Eggs, beaten – 3
Breakfast sausage, cooked and cooled – 1 pound
Cream cheese softened – 4 ounces
Coconut flour - .33 cup
Baking powder - .5 teaspoon
Sea salt – .5 teaspoon
Garlic powder - .5 teaspoon
Chives, dried – 3 tablespoons

The Instructions:
- Preheat your oven to a temperature of three-hundred and fifty degrees Fahrenheit while you prepare your breakfast sausage and allow it to slightly cool. Prepare a large cooking sheet by greasing it with oil or butter.
- In a medium-sized bowl, combine together the softened cream cheese and cooled sausage with a spoon, until the two are fully combined, and there are no cream cheese clumps remaining.
- Add the beaten egg, garlic powder, sea salt, dried chives, coconut flour, and baking powder to the cream cheese mixture, combining all of the

ingredients until they are fully incorporated. Place it in the fridge and allow it to chill for ten minutes. Do not skip this step.

- Use a small cookie scoop (which should be two tablespoons in volume) and create small balls of the mixture, placing them on the prepared baking pan each an inch apart.
- Place the baking pan in the oven and cook your breakfast bites until golden-brown and set about twenty minutes. Serve immediately or store in the fridge and enjoy either cold or reheated.

Cream Cheese Pancakes

These pancakes are decadent with their cream cheese and almond flour base. You will love them with Lakanto's maple-flavored syrup; warm berry compote; freshly whipped cream and strawberries; or even with bacon, eggs, and cheese sandwich between them. However, you serve these pancakes, they are sure to please a crowd.

The Details:
The Number of Servings: 3
The Time Needed to Prepare: 10
The Time Required to Cook: 5
The Total Preparation/Cook Time: 15
Number of Calories in Individual Servings: 271
Protein Grams: 9
Fat Grams: 25
Total Carbohydrates Grams: 3.5
Net Carbohydrates Grams: 2.5

The Ingredients:
Eggs – 4
Cream cheese softened – 4 ounces
Almond flour – 3 tablespoons
Lakanto sweetener – 2 teaspoons
Sea salt - .125 teaspoon
Butter, melted – 2 tablespoons
Lakanto Maple-Flavored Syrup (Optional)

The Instructions:
- In a blender, combine the eggs, cream cheese, almond flour, sweetener, and sea salt to create a thin batter.
- Heat your griddle over medium heat and add some of the melted butter to the pan. Using a tablespoon, form your pancake in the pan. Each pancake should contain two tablespoons worth of batter. The griddle should be hot enough that the pancakes immediately begin to cook once they hit the skillet. You will know it's hot enough when water sizzles and evaporates when drops are added to the pan.
- Cook each side of the pancakes for about one minute before flipping and cooking the other side. Remove the pancakes, add more butter and batter to the pan, and enjoy.

Creamy Parmesan Noodles

These noodles are the perfect low-carb alternative to your favorite pasta. You will find that the cream cheese creates a decadent sauce with Parmesan, garlic, and lemon zest. To make these noodles, you can use a vegetable spiralizer or simply make large flat noodles with a hand-held vegetable peeler.

The Details:

The Number of Servings: 2
The Time Needed to Prepare: 3 minutes
The Time Required to Cook: 5 minutes
The Total Preparation/Cook Time: 8 minutes
Number of Calories in Individual Servings: 247
Protein Grams: 8
Fat Grams: 19
Total Carbohydrates Grams: 12
Net Carbohydrates Grams: 10

The Ingredients:

Zucchini squash, medium, spiralized into noodles – 4
Parmesan cheese, grated - .25 cup
Cream cheese – 4 ounces
Garlic, minced – 4 cloves
Butter – 1 tablespoon
Sea salt – 1.5 teaspoons
Black pepper, ground - .25 teaspoon
Lemon zest - .5 teaspoon

The Instructions:

- Add the butter to a large skillet over medium heat and allow it to melt before adding in the garlic. Cook the garlic in the butter for a minute until it becomes fragrant.
- Once the garlic has cooked add the cream cheese, lemon zest, sea salt, and black ground pepper to the mix. Stir the sauce until the cream cheese melts into the butter. Add the zucchini noodles and Parmesan cheese, tossing them in the cream sauce.
- Continue to cook the noodles for a few minutes, just until the noodles are fork-tender. Serve and enjoy while still warm!

Chicken BLT Lettuce Wraps

These BLT wraps are better than your average BLT, as they are paired with creamy avocado and Ranch dressing. Whether you are enjoying these for an easy lunch or dinner, you will find that you can prepare these incredibly quickly if you keep some cooked chicken in the fridge ready to go.

The Details:
The Number of Servings: 3
The Time Needed to Prepare:
The Time Required to Cook:
The Total Preparation/Cook Time:
Number of Calories in Individual Servings: 346
Protein Grams: 22
Fat Grams: 24
Total Carbohydrates Grams: 13
Net Carbohydrates Grams: 8

The Ingredients:
Chicken thighs, boneless and skinless – 2
Avocado, diced - .5
Large tomato, diced - .5
Bacon, cooked, and chopped – 6 slices
Cilantro, chopped - .25 cup
Sea salt – .5 teaspoon
Black pepper, ground - .25 teaspoon
Iceberg or Boston Bibb lettuce – 1 head
Ranch dressing - .25 cup

The Instructions:
- Season your chicken with sea salt and black pepper, and then cook it on a grill in the oven set to three-hundred and seventy-five degrees Fahrenheit, or you can slice it and cook it on a skillet. However, you choose to cook your chicken, ensure that the center of it reaches one-hundred and sixty-five degrees Fahrenheit.
- Once the chicken is done cooking, allow it to rest at room temperature for ten minutes before slicing so that the juices remain intact within the meat. After you slice it, toss the chicken with the cilantro.
- While the chicken cools prepare your vegetables. You want to carefully remove each leaf of lettuce so that it stays intact in a boat or bowl shape.
- To create your wraps, layer the chicken, bacon, vegetables, and ranch in the lettuce cups. Serve immediately.

Cheeseburger Wraps

These cheeseburgers have all the fixings, and you will find that with fresh ingredients, they taste much better than anything you could get at a fast-food restaurant. You will never miss the bun, as these are full of flavor and decadence!

The Details:
The Number of Servings: 3
The Time Needed to Prepare: 5 minutes
The Time Required to Cook: 8 minutes
The Total Preparation/Cook Time: 13 minutes
Number of Calories in Individual Servings: 427
Protein Grams: 34
Fat Grams: 26
Total Carbohydrates Grams: 13
Net Carbohydrates Grams: 10

The Ingredients:
Cheddar cheese – 3 slices
Ground beef, 80/20% – .66 pound
Tomato, large, sliced – 1
Onion, small, thinly sliced – 1
Iceberg lettuce – 1 head
Sea salt - .5 teaspoon
Black pepper, ground - .25 teaspoon
Oregano, dried - .5 teaspoon
Mustard – 3 teaspoons
Ketchup – 3 teaspoons
Dill pickle relish – 3 teaspoons

The Instructions:
- Place a large skillet on the stove and allow it to preheat over medium heat. While it heats up, lightly combine the ground beef with the sea salt, black pepper, and oregano, being careful to not over mix or handle the meat. After the seasonings are combined into the meat, divide it into thirds and form each third into an individual patty.
- Place your patties on the skillet and allow each side to cook until browned, about three to four minutes on each side.
- While the burgers cook, prepare your vegetables.
- To assemble your burgers, take a few leaves of lettuce for each burger, divide the head between the three servings, and place the patty in the

middle of the leaves. On top of the patty, add your cheese, mustard, ketchup, and dill relish before topping it off with your onion and tomato slices. Fold the edges of the lettuce over the top of the burger patty to enclose it completely.

Creamy Broccoli Salad

This broccoli salad is creamy and savory, and you will find that even people who only tolerate broccoli love this salad. The cheese, roasted pumpkin seeds, and dressing perfectly compliment the salad. While most salads must be eaten immediately after assembly, this one can be made up to a day in advance, making it incredibly easy to take on the go and share with a crowd.

The Details:
The Number of Servings: 4
The Time Needed to Prepare: 5 minutes
The Time Required to Cook: 0 minutes
The Total Preparation/Cook Time: 5 minutes
Number of Calories in Individual Servings: 246
Protein Grams: 9
Fat Grams: 20
Total Carbohydrates Grams: 8
Net Carbohydrates Grams: 5

The Ingredients:
Broccoli florets, chopped into small pieces – 4 cups
Bacon, cooked, and chopped – 4 slices
Cheddar cheese, shredded - .5 cup
Red onion, diced - .5 cup
Pumpkin seeds, roasted - .25 cup
Apple cider vinegar – 1 tablespoon
Monk fruit sweetener – 1.5 tablespoons
Mayonnaise - .5 cup
Sea salt - .5 teaspoons

The Instructions:
- In a large salad bowl, whisk together the sea salt, monk fruit sweetener, apple cider vinegar, and mayonnaise. Add in the remaining ingredients and toss them all together until the broccoli is well coated.
- Cover the salad bowl and allow it to chill for at least an hour before serving, but it can be made up to a day in advance. You will find that the longer you chill the salad before serving, the better it will taste as the flavors will have more time to meld together.

Parmesan Garlic Roasted Green Beans

These green beans are the perfect side dish for any meal. Not only are they nutritious, but they are incredibly delicious, as well! The Parmesan and garlic pair perfectly with the fresh beans, which are then highlighted by the toasted almonds.

The Details:
The Number of Servings: 4
The Time Needed to Prepare: 5 minutes
The Time Required to Cook: 2o minutes
The Total Preparation/Cook Time: 25 minutes
Number of Calories in Individual Servings: 145
Protein Grams: 4
Fat Grams: 11
Total Carbohydrates Grams: 9
Net Carbohydrates Grams: 6

The Ingredients:
Green beans, fresh – 1 pound
Olive oil – 2 tablespoons
Parmesan cheese, grated – 2 tablespoons
Sliced almonds, toasted - .25 cup
Sea salt - .5 teaspoon
Garlic powder - .25 teaspoon

The Instructions:
- Preheat your oven to a temperature of four-hundred degrees Fahrenheit and prepare a large baking sheet for the green beans.
- In a large bowl, toss together the green beans and olive oil. Sprinkle the Parmesan cheese, sea salt, and garlic powder over the top and toss again until the green beans are evenly coated in the seasonings. Spread the green beans over the prepared baking pan and set it in the oven.
- Bake the green beans for twenty minutes, stirring them once halfway through the cooking time. When you remove the pan from the oven, sprinkle the toasted almonds over the top before serving.

Dill Pickle Snack Rolls

These rolls are quick, easy, and only require a handful of ingredients. With these dill pickle snack rolls, you can get a quick protein-and-fat fix, allowing you to up your energy and stay sustained until your next mealtime.

The Details:
The Number of Servings: 2
The Time Needed to Prepare: 2 minutes
The Time Required to Cook: 0 minutes
The Total Preparation/Cook Time: 2 minutes
Number of Calories in Individual Servings: 189
Protein Grams: 12
Fat Grams: 13
Total Carbohydrates Grams: 5
Net Carbohydrates Grams: 4

The Ingredients:
Dill pickles, mini – 4
Sandwich ham – 4 slices
Cream cheese – 4 tablespoons
Everything Bagel seasoning – 2 teaspoons

The Instructions:
- Lay the four slices of ham out side-by-side. Spread one tablespoon of cream cheese over the top of each slice and then sprinkle the Bagel seasoning over the cream cheese.
- Place one mini dill pickle on top of each slice of ham and cream cheese, and then tightly roll them so that the pickle is wrapped in the ham and cheese. Serve whole or slice them into rounds before enjoying.

Bacon Deviled Eggs

These deviled eggs are salty and smokey from the bacon and smoked paprika, which is perfectly complemented with the light Dijon and the fresh chives. These are a great snack to keep in the fridge at all times, as you can simply grab a serving whenever you need a snack or don't have time to prepare a meal.

The Details:
The Number of Servings: 3
The Time Needed to Prepare: 25 minutes
The Time Required to Cook: 10 minutes
The Total Preparation/Cook Time: 35 minutes
Number of Calories in Individual Servings: 239
Protein Grams: 14
Fat Grams: 19
Total Carbohydrates Grams: 1
Net Carbohydrates Grams: 1

The Ingredients:
Eggs, large – 6
Mayonnaise - .25 cup
Chives, chopped – 1 tablespoon
Dijon mustard – 1 teaspoon
Sea salt - .25 teaspoon
Smoked paprika - .25 teaspoon
Bacon cooked and crumbled – 2 slices

The Instructions:
- Place the eggs in a large saucepan and cover them completely with water so that the water raises about one and a half inches over the top of the eggs. Bring the water to a rolling boil, remove from the heat, and allow the eggs to sit in the water for fifteen minutes.
- When the eggs are done sitting, pour off the water, rinse them in cool water, and then place them in an ice-water bath to chill for five minutes.
- Peel the eggs and then cut them in half length-wise. Use a spoon and gently remove the yolks from the eggs, placing the yolks in a small bowl and the egg whites on a large plate.
- Use a fork and mash the egg yolks completely and then mix in the remaining ingredients until it forms a creamy mixture. Use a spoon and scoop the egg yolk mixture back into the center of the eggs. Serve immediately or chill in the fridge for up to two days before eating.

Toll House-Style Chocolate Chip Cookies

Just because you are eating healthy doesn't mean you can't have dessert! These cookies make use of popular low-carb baking ingredients such as Lakanto brand sweetener and Lily's stevia-sweetened baking chocolate chips. You will absolutely love these cookies and find that they please everyone, from children to adults.

The Details:
The Number of Servings: 15
The Time Needed to Prepare: 10 minutes
The Time Required to Cook: 10 minutes
The Total Preparation/Cook Time: 20 minutes
Number of Calories in Individual Servings: 215
Protein Grams: 4
Fat Grams: 20
Total Carbohydrates Grams: 9
Net Carbohydrates Grams: 2.65

The Ingredients:
Coconut oil, melted - .25 cup
Butter softened - .5 cup
Egg – 1
Lakanto golden monk fruit sweetener - .25 cup
Lakanto classic monk fruit sweetener - .33 cup
Almond extract - .5 teaspoon
Vanilla extract – 1 teaspoon
Sea salt – .5 teaspoon
Baking soda - .5 teaspoon
Almond flour – 2 cups
Coconut flour – 2 tablespoons
Lily's dark chocolate chips – 1 cup

The Instructions:
- Preheat your oven cooking device to a temperature of three-hundred and fifty degrees Fahrenheit before laying a sheet of kitchen parchment on a large baking pan.
- In a bowl that is medium in size, whip together the softened butter and melted coconut oil. Add in both Lakanto sweeteners, coconut flour, the egg, and the flavor extracts.
- In another bowl, combine the baking soda, sea salt, and almond flour. Once the dry ingredients are well incorporated, add them into the bowl

with the wet ingredients and mix all of the ingredients together until it is light and fluffy.

- Fold in Lily's stevia-sweetened chocolate chips.
- Roll the cookie dough into thirty small dough balls and then place them on the baking pan each ½-inch apart. Press down the dough slightly with your fingers so that they are all circular cookie shapes.
- Place the cookie pan in the middle of your oven and bake until the cookies are golden and set for 10 minutes. Allow the cookies to cool for a few minutes before eating so that they do not crumble or fall apart.

Mascarpone Brownies

These flourless brownies are gooey and delicious, with the mascarpone cheese offering a wonderful flavor and texture. But, if you can not get your hands on mascarpone cheese that is okay! Instead, you can always use a mixture of half cream cheese and half sour cream. Whether you use authentic mascarpone cheese or the cream cheese/sour cream substitute, you will find that these brownies are absolutely delicious.

The Details:
The Number of Servings: 10
The Time Needed to Prepare: 10 minutes
The Time Required to Cook: 25 minutes
The Total Preparation/Cook Time: 35 minutes
Number of Calories in Individual Servings: 148
Protein Grams: 2.75
Fat Grams: 12
Total Carbohydrates Grams: 10
Net Carbohydrates Grams: 2.5

The Ingredients:
Eggs – 3
Mascarpone cheese - .25 cup
Butter, melted - .25 cup
Cocoa powder - .25 cup
Lily's dark chocolate chips – 1 cup
Lakanto Monk fruit sweetener - .75 cup
Sea salt - .5 teaspoon
Vanilla extract – 1 teaspoon

The Instructions:
- Preheat your oven to a temperature of three-hundred and seventy-five degrees Fahrenheit. Using kitchen parchment, line an eight-inch by eight-inch square baking pan.
- In the microwave, melt the butter and chocolate chips together in a small glass bowl, stirring it every 30 seconds until melted. Once melted, stir the two ingredients together again until they are completely combined.
- In a medium-size bowl for the purpose of mixing, beat together the Lakanto sweetener and eggs for three to four minutes, until fluffy. Add in the mascarpone cheese and beat for an additional minute before beating in the cocoa powder. The mixture should be creamy and smooth when you are done.

- Pour the butter and melted chocolate mixture into the mascarpone cheese batter and beat the mixture together until fully incorporated. Spread this mixture into your prepared brownie pan that is lined with kitchen parchment.
- Place the brownie pan in the oven and allow it to cook for twenty-five minutes, and then allow it to cool at room temperature for ten minutes before slicing or serving.

Strawberry Shortcake

These strawberry shortcakes offer the ideal decadent whipped cream, sweet and tangy fresh strawberries, and a delicious almond cake. While this dessert may be decadent, it is incredibly easy to make. You will be able to thoroughly enjoy this dessert, as will any guests you serve it to.

The Details:

The Number of Servings: 10
The Time Needed to Prepare: 15 minutes
The Time Required to Cook: 15 minutes
The Total Preparation/Cook Time: 30 minutes
Number of Calories in Individual Servings: 201
Protein Grams: 4
Fat Grams: 18
Total Carbohydrates Grams: 6.5
Net Carbohydrates Grams: 4.5

The Ingredients:

Butter, melted – 6 tablespoons
Egg whites – 5
Cream of tartar - .5 teaspoon
Lakanto sweetener - .33 cup
Vanilla extract - .5 teaspoon
Baking powder – 1.5 teaspoon
Coconut flour - .5 tablespoon
Almond flour – 1 cup
Sea salt - .25 teaspoon
Heavy whipping cream - .75 cup
Lakanto sweetener – 4 tablespoons
Strawberries, hulled and sliced – 1 pound

The Instructions:

- Preheat your oven to a temperature of three-hundred and fifty degrees Fahrenheit. Place ten paper liners in a muffin tin and set it aside while you prepare your shortcakes.
- In a clean large mixing bowl, beat the egg whites and cream of tartar on high speed until the egg white form shiny stiff peaks. Once the stiff peaks have formed, slowly pour the melted butter into the mixture and beat it at low speed. Add in the sweetener and vanilla just until combined.
- In a different mixing bowl, combine the sea salt, coconut flour, baking powder, and almond flour until all of the ingredients are combined.

- Gently fold the almond flour mixture into the egg white mixture until it is fully combined. Divide this batter between the ten lined muffin cups and bake in the oven until the edges have turned golden-brown for about fifteen minutes.
- Once the shortcakes are done cooking, allow them to cool down and prepare the toppings. To do this wash, hull, and slice the strawberries. Toss the strawberries in one of the four tablespoons of Lakanto sweetener and then set them aside.
- Place the whipped cream in a clean bowl and whip it until it forms soft peaks. Add in the remaining three tablespoons of Lakanto sweetener and beat the cream for an additional minute.
- To serve, remove the shortcakes from the paper liners and place each one on a serving plate. Top the shortcakes with the whipped cream and strawberries on top.

Italian Cream Cake

While you can certainly make plenty of quick and easy keto desserts, sometimes, we want something fancy or something that will feed a crowd. For times like those, you can do no better than this creamy and nutty Italian cream cake. Whether it is your birthday, Christmas, or simply another day of the week, you will love this decadent treat.

The Details:

The Number of Servings: 12
The Time Needed to Prepare:
The Time Required to Cook:
The Total Preparation/Cook Time:
Number of Calories in Individual Servings: 423
Protein Grams: 7
Fat Grams: 42
Total Carbohydrates Grams: 6
Net Carbohydrates Grams: 4

The Cake Ingredients:

Eggs, large, at room temperature – 4
Butter softened - .5 cup
Heavy cream - .5 cup
Lakanto Monk fruit sweetener – 1 cup
Vanilla extract – 1 teaspoon
Almond flour – 1.5 cups
coconut flour - .25 cup
Sea salt - .5 teaspoon
Baking powder – 2 teaspoons
Cream of tartar - .25 teaspoon
Pecans, chopped - .5 cup
Coconut, unsweetened, shredded - .5 cup

The Frosting Ingredients:

Butter softened - .5 cup
Cream cheese, room temperature – 8 ounces
Heavy cream - .5 cup
Powdered Swerve sweetener – 1 cup
Coconut, unsweetened, toasted – 2 tablespoons
Pecans, chopped, toasted – 2 tablespoons

The Instructions:

- Preheat your oven to a temperature of three-hundred and twenty-five degrees Fahrenheit and prepare your cake pans. You will need to line the bottom of six nine-inch round cake pans and then grease them.
- In a large bowl for the purpose of mixing, whisk together the almond flour, coconut flour, sea salt, baking powder, pecans, and coconut from the set of cake ingredients. Once they are combined, set the bowl aside.
- In a medium kitchen bowl, beat together the softened butter and Lakanto monk fruit sweetener with a hand beater for about two minutes until it is light and fluffy.
- Separate the eggs, ensuring that no bits of yolk or any other fat come into contact with the egg whites. A single drop of fat from egg yolks or another source will prevent the egg whites from beating into peaks.
- Place the eggs one at a time into the butter and sweetener mixture, beating well after each addition of egg yolk so that it is completely incorporated into the butter. Beat in the heavy cream and vanilla extract.
- In a separate large and completely dry and clean kitchen bowl, beat the egg whites with the cream of tartar until they form stiff peaks that can stand on their own.
- Using a rubber spatula, gently fold the egg whites into the cake batter. Be sure to do this slowly and carefully so that the egg whites retain their integrity and lighten the cake batter.
- Divide the batter between the six cake pans, and then place them in the oven to cook until the center of the cake is firm and the edges are a beautiful golden color about thirty-five to forty minutes.
- Remove the cakes from the oven and allow them to cool completely in the pans. Once cooled, carefully remove the cakes from the pans.
- After the cakes are fully cooled and removed from their pans, begin to prepare the frosting. To do this, first cream the softened cream cheese and butter together with a kitchen beater until fluffy, about two minutes.
- Beat the vanilla and powdered Swerve sweetener into creamed mixture, and then slowly add the heavy cream until the frosting reaches your preferred thickness. You can add either more or less cream if you desire.
- Spread some of the frostings over two of the cake layers. Place one of these layers on a platter and then set the remaining layers on top with the other frosted layer on the very top of all the other layers. Once your layers are all stacked up, frost the sides of the cake with the remaining frosting.
- Sprinkle the toasted coconut and pecans over the cake before slicing. Serve the cake at room temperature or chilled.

Key Lime Curd Bars

These key lime curd bars offer a sweet tang which is perfectly complemented with the shortbread cookie crust. Served chilled, these bars are incredibly refreshing and can be enjoyed year-round. Whether you are enjoying them for a cold summer treat or a decadent dessert during the holidays, you will love them year-round.

The Details:
The Number of Servings: 12
The Time Needed to Prepare: 10 minutes
The Time Required to Cook: 40 minutes
The Total Preparation/Cook Time: 50 minutes
Number of Calories in Individual Servings: 289
Protein Grams: 6
Fat Grams: 28
Total Carbohydrates Grams: 4.5
Net Carbohydrates Grams: 2.5

The Ingredients:
Eggs, large – 8
Lakanto Monk fruit sweetener - .75 cup
Coconut oil, melted – 1 cup
Key lime juice - .75 cup
Almond flour – 1.5 cups
Coconut flour - .5 cup
Sea salt - .25 teaspoon
Baking powder – 1 teaspoon
Lakanto Monk fruit sweetener – 1 cup

The Instructions:

- Preheat your oven to a temperature of Fahrenheit three-hundred and twenty-five degrees, and prepare an eight-by-eight-inch glass baking pan by greasing it with butter or coconut oil.

- In a small bowl, combine together the coconut oil and Lakanto three-quarters of a cup of sweetener. Once combined, add in the coconut flour, almond flour, and sea salt using a kitchen hand beater. Press this into the bottom of the pan with your hands to form a thin crust.

- Place the crust in the oven and allow it to bake until a pale golden-brown, about fifteen minutes. Allow it to cool at room temperature.

- In a blender, combine the baking powder, sea salt, key lime juice, one cup of Lakanto sweetener, and eight eggs until completely smooth. Spread this mixture over the top of the cooled pre-cooked crust.
- Place the pan in the preheated oven and cook until the filling has turned a light golden color and the middle has set up for about thirty-five to forty minutes.
- If the top of the bars begins to turn overly dark and the middle is not yet set, then you can cover it with aluminum foil during the remainder of the cooking process.
- Allow the bars to come to room temperature and then place it in the fridge to set until cold. Slice and serve the bars once cold and for up to five days after cooking.

Thin Mint Cookies

It can be hard to pass up the many Girl Scout cookie choices every season, especially when they are being sold door-to-door and in front of every major grocery store. But, you don't have to let these high-carb sugary confections ruin your weight and good health, not when you can make your own! If you like chocolate mints, then you will love these thin mints.

The Details:

The Number of Servings: 15
The Time Needed to Prepare:
The Time Required to Cook:
The Total Preparation/Cook Time:
Number of Calories in Individual Servings: 152
Protein Grams: 3
Fat Grams: 8
Total Carbohydrates Grams: 11
Net Carbohydrates Grams: 2.5

The Ingredients:

Egg, large, beaten – 1
Butter, melted – 2 tablespoons
Lakanto Monk fruit sweetener - .33 cup
Sea salt - .25 teaspoon
Baking powder – 1 teaspoon
Vanilla extract - .5 teaspoon
Cocoa powder - .33 cup
Almond flour – 1.75 cups
Lily's dark chocolate chips – 7 ounces
Coconut oil – 1 tablespoon
Peppermint extract – 1 teaspoon

The Instructions:

- Preheat your oven to a temperature of Fahrenheit three-hundred degrees and line two baking sheets with kitchen parchment.
- In a mixing bowl, stir together the baking powder, sea salt, Lakanto sweetener, cocoa powder, and almond flour. Once combined, stir in melted butter, egg, and vanilla extract until it forms a thick dough.
- Place the dough on a piece of kitchen parchment or wax-coated paper and place an additional sheet on top of the dough, so that the dough is sandwiched between the two pieces of paper. Using a rolling pin, roll the dough out until it is one-quarter of an inch thick and no thicker.

Carefully peel the top piece of paper off of the rolled cookie dough and discard.

- Using a cookie cutter that is round and two inches in diameter, cut the dough into small rounds. Gently lift the cut-out cookies with either your hands or a spatula and place them on the prepared cookie sheets each half an inch apart.

- Bake the cookies until they are firm, about twenty to thirty minutes. The exact time will depend on how thinly you rolled out your dough.

- Once the cookies are done cooking, remove them from the pan and allow them to cool on a wire kitchen rack.

- After the cookies have cooled, begin to prepare the chocolate. To do this, bring a saucepan of water to a gentle simmer and set a metal bowl over the top of the pot. You don't want the water to touch the bowl. This will create a double boiler.

- Add the chocolate to the bowl portion of the double boiler and continue to stir it until it is fully melted. Remove the chocolate from the heat and then stir in the peppermint extract.

- One at a time, place the cookies in the chocolate and use a set of two forks to adjust coat each cookie in the mint chocolate. Lift the cookie out of the chocolate, gently tapping the fork against the side of the bowl to allow any excess chocolate to drip off.

- Once you coat each cookie, place it on a kitchen parchment or wax-coated paper-lined pan. Once the pan is full of cookies, place it in the fridge and allow the thin mints to chill until the chocolate is fully set.

- After the chocolate has been set, you can store the cookies at room temperature, in the fridge, or in the freezer.

Pumpkin Pie Cheesecake Bars

Whether you love cheesecake, pumpkin pie, or pumpkin spice lattes, you will find that these bars are the perfect autumn treat! Enjoy them for a simple day of autumn baking, or celebrate your Thanksgiving feast with these bars. You can enjoy and celebrate Thanksgiving without gaining weight or overloading on sugar and carbs.

The Details:
The Number of Servings: 8
The Time Needed to Prepare: 15 minutes
The Time Required to Cook: 60 minutes
The Total Preparation/Cook Time: 75 minutes
Number of Calories in Individual Servings: 324
Protein Grams: 7
Fat Grams: 31
Total Carbohydrates Grams: 6
Net Carbohydrates Grams: 4

The Ingredients:
Cream cheese softened – 16 ounces
Eggs, large – 2
Pumpkin, canned – .5 cup
Butter, melted – 3 tablespoons
Powdered Swerve sweetener - .75 cup plus 1 tablespoon
Almond flour – 1 cup
Cinnamon, ground - .5 teaspoon
Cloves, ground – pinch
Ginger, ground - .25 teaspoon
Sea salt - .25 teaspoon

The Instructions:
- Preheat your oven to a temperature of Fahrenheit three hundred degrees and prepare a square eight-by-eight inch baking dish covering both the bottom and sides with kitchen parchment.
- In a small bowl, combine the melted butter, one tablespoon of Swerve sweetener, sea salt, and almond flour until they are fully integrated with each other. Pour this mixture into your prepared dish and use your fingers to flatten it into an even and smooth crust.
- Bake the crust in the preheated oven until it is set and golden, about twelve minutes. Remove it from the oven, and allow it to cool for at least ten minutes while you prepare the remainder of the components.

- Increase your oven temperature to Fahrenheit three-hundred and fifty degrees.
- In a large bowl, beat together the remaining Swerve sweetener and the cream cheese until it is light and fluffy, about a minute or two with an electric hand beater. Add in the eggs one at a time, beating well after each addition.
- Pour half of this cream cheese mixture over the pre-baked crust and spread it out into a flat layer.
- Into the remaining half of the cream cheese mixture that is still in your bowl, add in the spices and pumpkin, beating them again until light and fluffy.
- Gently and carefully spoon the pumpkin mixture over the layer of cream cheese mixture, and then spread it out into an even layer over the cream cheese layer. You want to do this carefully so that you do not disturb the cream cheese layer underneath.
- Bake your bars until they have set, about forty to forty-five minutes. Once done cooking, remove it from the oven and allow it to cool at room temperature.
- Once the bars have cooled, place the pan in the fridge and let it chill overnight before slicing and serving. Serve alone or with some freshly whipped cream.

Better-Than-Reese's Almond Butter Cups

These almond butter cups are to die for! Of course, if you prefer peanut butter, you can use a sugar-free variety instead of almond butter. You might also try sprinkling them with some coarse sea salt over the top of the chocolate, or using crunchy nut butter instead of smooth. As you can see, there are many variations you can make in order to attain your ideal nut buttercup.

The Details:
The Number of Servings: 10
The Time Needed to Prepare: 10 minutes
The Time Required to Cook: 2 minutes
The Total Preparation/Cook Time: 12 minutes
Number of Calories in Individual Servings: 320
Protein Grams: 7
Fat Grams: 28
Total Carbohydrates Grams: 20
Net Carbohydrates Grams: 4

The Ingredients:
Almond butter, sugar-free – 1 cup
Powdered Swerve sweetener - .25 cup
Lily's dark chocolate chips – 10 ounces
Coconut oil, melted – 4 tablespoons, divided

The Instructions:
- In the microwave, place the dark chocolate chips and two tablespoons of coconut oil in a glass bowl. Melt the chocolate, stirring it every thirty seconds until fully melted. The time needed to melt the chocolate can vary greatly depending on your individual microwave and its settings.
- Place silicone molds on a baking sheet. You can use any silicone mold that has mostly flat surfaces, such as egg-shaped molds or muffin molds. Avoid molds that have a variety of shapes or textures, such as animal molds. My favorite to use is muffin cup molds, as these make the traditional nut butter cup shape.
- Spoon a small amount of the melted chocolate into the bottom of each silicone cup. You want enough chocolate to coat both the bottom and the sides. Use a silicone pastry brush to brush the chocolate up the sides of the cup for an even coating.
- Place your chocolate cups in the freezer for fifteen minutes, until the chocolate hardens.

- While the chocolate is in the freezer, combine the almond butter, powdered Swerve sweetener, and the remaining two tablespoons of melted coconut oil until it is smooth and evenly distributed.
- After the chocolate has hardened, divide the almond butter between the chocolate cups and then cover the nut butter mixture with the remaining chocolate.
- Place the cups in the freezer for an additional fifteen minutes to harden before storing the cups in the fridge.

Blueberry Crumble Bars

This delicious blueberry crumble bars are reminiscent of fruit and oat bars, but without all the carbs! The almonds and coconut make an ideal replacement for the oats, as they not only have a fun texture, but also have a delicious flavor perfect for complimenting berries. If you don't care for blueberries, then you can try making these bars with other berry options!

The Details:
The Number of Servings: 6
The Time Needed to Prepare: 10 minutes
The Time Required to Cook: 35 minutes
The Total Preparation/Cook Time: 45 minutes
Number of Calories in Individual Servings: 297
Protein Grams: 5
Fat Grams: 27
Total Carbohydrates Grams: 10
Net Carbohydrates Grams: 6

The Ingredients:
Blueberries – 1 cup
Xanthan gum - .25 teaspoon
Powdered Swerve sweetener - .25 cup
Water – 2 tablespoons
Coconut flour – 2 tablespoons
Coconut, shredded, unsweetened - .75 cup
Almond flour – 1.5 cups
Lakanto Monk fruit sweetener - .5 cup
Vanilla extract – .5 teaspoon
Almond extract - .5 teaspoon
Sea salt - .5 teaspoon
Butter, melted – 6 tablespoons

The Instructions:
- Preheat your oven to a temperature of Fahrenheit three-hundred and fifty degrees and prepare an eight-by-eight-inch square baking dish by lining it with kitchen parchment.
- Place the blueberries and water in a kitchen pot over a temperature of medium-high heat. Bring the water to a simmer and allow the berries to cook until they are softened.

- Mash the blueberries slightly and then vigorously whisk in the powdered Swerve sweetener and xanthan gum. Allow the blueberry mixture to cool, and as it does, the xanthan gum will thicken the liquid.
- In a medium-sized bowl for the purpose of mixing, combine the Lakanto monk fruit sweetener, shredded coconut, coconut flour, almond flour, and sea salt. Add in the vanilla extract, almond extract, and melted butter, stirring the mixture together until it forms clumps.
- Divide the dough into two portions and place one of the portions into your prepared baking dish. Using your fingers, press the dough firmly and evenly into the bottom of the pan.
- Bake the crust in the pan for ten minutes and then allow it to cool for ten more minutes. Once cooled, spread the blueberry mixture over the top and crumble the remaining crust mixture over the top of the blueberries. Lightly press on the crumble topping so that it sticks to the blueberry mixture.
- Place the pan back in the oven and cook until the crumble has turned golden and the blueberry mixture is bubbling, about twenty to twenty-five minutes.
- Remove the pan from the oven and allow it to cool completely before slicing or serving. Store the bars in the fridge.

No-Bake Cheesecake

This cheesecake is full of flavor and has the most luscious and creamy texture. You will love the way it tastes, either on its own or with your favorite berries or chocolate. It is best to prepare this cheesecake the day before you intend to serve it, just to make sure that if the temperature of your fridge is off that it is fully set up before cutting.

The Details:
The Number of Servings: 12
The Time Needed to Prepare: 10 minutes
The Time Required to Chill: 5 hours
The Total Preparation/Chill Time: 5 Hours, 10 Minutes
Number of Calories in Individual Servings: 337
Protein Grams: 6
Fat Grams: 12
Total Carbohydrates Grams: 5
Net Carbohydrates Grams: 4

The Ingredients:
Almond flour – 2 cups
Melted butter - .33 cup
Powdered Swerve sweetener – 3 tablespoons
Vanilla extract – 1.5 teaspoons
Cream cheese softened – 16 ounces
Sour cream - .5 cup
Heavy cream - .75 cup
Powdered Swerve sweetener – 1 cup

The Instructions:
- In a bowl, combine the three tablespoons of powdered Swerve sweetener, almond flour, melted butter, and half of a teaspoon of vanilla extract. Press this mixture into the bottom of a nine-inch pie plate and then allow it to chill for at least one hour.
- In a large bowl and using an electric beater, combine the softened cream cheese, one teaspoon of vanilla extract, and one cup of powdered Swerve sweetener until the mixture is light, fluffy, and creamy.
- Add the heavy cream and sour cream into the cream cheese mixture and continue to beat until it develops a texture reminiscent of pudding. Pour the mixture into the chilled pie crust, using a rubber spatula to smooth out the top.

- Place the cheesecake in the fridge and allow it to chill for at least four hours or overnight before slicing.

Conclusion

Thank you for finishing *Keto for Women over 50*! I hope that this book has given you everything you need to know to gain health, increase energy, reduce weight loss, and decrease your risk of developing diseases. As no person exists inside a vacuum, neither does our health. For this reason, gender and age can play a role in affecting our health and keto journey. Thankfully, as you have learned in this book, the ketogenic diet is especially helpful for women fifty and older.

No matter your background, you no longer have to worry about your weight, health, and energy levels drastically altering from one year to the next. Instead, you can enjoy a comfortable and manageable weight, increases health, and an energy boost.

Many people go through their adulthood trying one crash and fad diet after the next, only for it to ruin their metabolism. You no longer have to struggle along with this frustrating roller coaster. There is an answer that is neither fad nor crash diet. Instead, the ketogenic diet was created by scientists for better health, and you can receive all those benefits.

By following the directions of this book and working alongside your doctor, you can soon gain everything that you have hoped for.

Thank you again for finishing this book! If you found it helpful please consider leaving a review online.

CPSIA information can be obtained
at www.ICGtesting.com
Printed in the USA
LVHW011308130621
690102LV00014B/2005